The 30-Day Total Health Makeover

Also by Marilu Henner

Marilu Henner's Total Health Makeover

By All Means Keep On Moving

I Refuse to Raise a Brat

Healthy Life Kitchen

The 30-Day
Total Health Makeover

Marilu Henner

with Laura Morton

ReganBooks

An Imprint of HarperCollins*Publishers*

To my family

> This book is not intended to replace medical advice or to be a substitute for a physician. Always seek the advice of a physician before beginning any diet and/or exercise program.
>
> The author and the publisher expressly disclaim responsibility for any adverse effects arising from following the diet or exercise program in this book without appropriate medical supervision.

Contents

Contents

Contents

Acknowledgments

Without the support, talent, and hard work from the following people, this project would never have been possible.

To Judith Regan, whose insight, expertise, and encouragement have given me a whole new career—her incredible team at Regan Books and HarperCollins, Amye Dyer, Joseph Mills, Robin Arzt, Angelica Canales, Rick Pracher, Steven Sorrentino, and especially Paul Olsewski who arranged the longest book tour in the history of publishing. (I can't wait to do it again!)

To Mel Berger, Marc Schwartz, Sam Haskell, Rick Bradley, and Jerry Katzman of the William Morris Agency, Dick Guttman and Susan Madore of Guttman & Associates, Richard Feldstein and Barbara Karrol at Provident Financial Management, Jill Brevda and Lois O'Hallaran of Intel, Charles Bush, and Sharon Feldstein, who always wins best dressed.

To all of the wonderful chefs who contributed their time and recipes to this book: Nina Andro, Jimmy Bradley, Elizabeth Carney, JoAnn Carney, Lance Correlez, Danny DeVito, Jane Downs and Mary Micucci, Mark C. Elliman, Serge Falesitch, Susan Feniger, Maggie Fountain, Martin Frost, Dale Greenblatt, Mary Ann Hennings, Louis Lanza, Lorne Lieberman, Robert Lieberman, Barbara J. Lloyd, Jeremy Marshall, Sorke Peters, Wolfgang Puck, James B. Reesor, Hans Rockenwagner, Joe Rowley, Leonard Schwartz, Joachim Splichal, and Isabel Williams. It just goes to show you that you *can*

Acknowledgments

eat well on this program. To Dr. Ted Pastrick and Dr. Tim Liddy for their professional contributions as well.

To Dr. Ruth Velikovsky Sharon, the brilliant psychoanalyst who has helped me clean up my mind clutter for many years.

To the world's greatest, smartest, funniest, and healthiest (after spending over 30 days with me) team. To Brent Strickland and his magic fingers and great attitude. To Trent Othick for never saying no. To Jim Sperber for finding what we needed three hours before we needed it. To Elizabeth Carney, who joined the team late but, as usual, saved the day. To Caroline Aaron, whose observational skills helped tap in to my creativity and gave this project a unique flavor. I never want to do a book without you. To my sister-in-law Lynnette—my MVP, who tirelessly shopped, read, researched, and tagged. (We're proud of her new title as Ms. Staples '99.) To my brother Lorin—who has worked on all four books with me. No one works harder or makes me laugh more than you do. (What exactly do you do again?) Seriously, you are a jack of all trades. And to Laura Morton—for her talent, inspiration, and contribution to this book.

To Elena Lewis, who kept everything organized despite the chaos the writing team wreaked all over the house.

To Donna Erickson, who once again made it possible for me to do my work knowing that my children were being well taken care of in the next room.

And to my guys, Rob, Nicky, and Joey, who remain the best reasons for living a long, happy, and healthy life.

Introduction

What an incredible year this has been! Since the release of my last book, *Marilu Henner's Total Health Makeover*, I have made nearly 300 appearances all over the country, which gave me the opportunity to talk to so many people. I've met people in airports, at book signings, in talk show waiting rooms, even at the Home Shopping Network! I've met people of all ages who want to get healthy. Older people who've been told by their doctors that they need to change their lifestyle. Baby boomers who would like to feel young and vibrant. People in their twenties who know enough about the current trends in nutrition to know that the old ways of thinking won't give them the answers. (I even met young kids who weren't born when *Taxi* went off the air, but watch the show on "Nick at Night" and just wanted to meet Nardo!) There was even a fifteen-year-old ballerina who said that the information in the book was saving her from anorexia. I met her in Nashville, and she told me that she was reading the book, and was learning how to battle her eating disorder. It was incredible talking to her. Two months later, I was in Tampa, giving a lecture to a group of young performers from Ann Reinking's Broadway Theater Project, and I decided to tell her story. Imagine my surprise when after my speech that same young girl came up to me and said, "I'm that ballerina you were talking about." She looked so much better. You could see a vibrancy in her face that wasn't there before.

I've met so many people who are looking for something beyond weight loss, which was really the message of *Total Health Makeover*—to get beyond thinking of "health" as losing weight in a quick temporary way.

With each and every appearance, there were so many people who were ready for the next step. I saw thousands of new faces eager to share their success stories with me and anxious to hear my answers to all of their questions. In the history of publishing, I don't think anyone has been given the opportunity to talk about a book as much as I did last year. But boy, am I glad I did, because after years of talking about it, I finally had the chance to make my dream of "getting the information out there" come true. And now that I've gotten us on the road of total health and well-being, it's time for us to share the next step together.

I received tens of thousands of letters, e-mails, and personal messages asking me all sorts of questions, but the number one request was for a 30-day plan that shows exactly what I do almost every day of my life. When that request kept coming up, it reminded me of my sisters and friends coming to my house and saying "I'm going to give myself over to your program!" My family and friends always joke that staying at my house is better than going to a spa. (I have one friend who comes to my house, opens the refrigerator, and screams because she doesn't recognize anything in it, although her husband says, "I've never had a bad meal at Marilu's.") By the time they all leave, however, they not only learn how to eat better and exercise more efficiently, but also how to organize their time better, use things around the house as part of their beauty routine, and—sometimes—how to "fake" feeling better even if they're having a bad day. When planning a 30-day program, I realized that all I had to do was treat everyone out there who wanted a specific plan as if they were a real guest in my home. It would be an open invitation to spend a month with me, Marilu. If you were to be a guest in my home for 30 days, the plan in this book is pretty much what you would take away from that experience—a total picture of healthy eating, exercising, and organization. Growing up in a large family with very little privacy taught me at a young age that life is all about organization (and boys and my weight, of course)! And it still is.

It's almost the next century, and life has become about streamlining because there just aren't enough hours in the day. Time is such a precious commodity—as precious as our health—and neither of them should be taken for granted. It's such a waste of time not being healthy. Who has the time, let alone the desire, to be sick? Under many circumstances, it's unnecessary and it's *always* a waste of our energy and spirit. If you can't make time for your health, you will have to make time for illness. With all the information that's out there we now know too much to ignore our health. But our health goes beyond what we put in our bodies. It is a mind-body-environment connection that can't be viewed separately.

If you're anything like me, every once in a while you have this need to start cleaning things out. You start in your closets and then move on to the drawers. You clean out your makeup bag, and then tackle that pile of mail that's been sitting forever. Before you know it, you're organized and ready for the next thing. But what I'm talking about is more than just cleaning up your living space. It's also about cleaning up your mind, your body, and your soul. You see, for me, being healthy isn't just about eliminating the junk from your body or from the food that you eat. It's also about eliminating the junk that clogs up your life. It's all part of the formula that brings you to the B.E.S.T. (Balance, Energy, Stamina, Toxin-Free) version of yourself—from the inside out, the outside in, and everywhere in between. It's not just about your weight, it's about your whole life picture. Because they're all part of the same thing. After all—*everything* is connected to everything.

When I was eight years old, I had a true epiphany. I was sitting in Sister Paula Marie's third grade class and we were taking a math test. One of the questions was "How many pencils are in a score?" And I thought to myself, "A score? What's a score? I've never even heard of a score." I panicked, because I didn't want to get a wrong answer on this test. I had to be able to figure it out. So I did all the other answers first, and I came back to this one and I thought, "Come on—you can do it." And suddenly, it came to me! I figured out how to figure it out. "Oh my gosh, I've heard of a score before. 'Four score and seven years ago.' Of course. The Gettysburg Address! Let's see—that was during the Civil War, and they were talking about the signing of the Declaration of Independence—and if I figure out how long ago that was, maybe I could figure out what a score is." And sure enough, I figured out that there were eighty-seven years between the two events. "Four score and seven years ago, eighty seven minus seven equals eighty, divided by four, is TWENTY!" And I remember thinking—*"Everything is connected to everything!"* I put my pencil down, and it was as if the heavens had parted and the angels were singing the Hallelujah Chorus. EVERY-THING IS CONNECTED TO EVERYTHING! The whole world opened up to me in that moment. What I learned in math was connected to history—history was connected to religion—religion was connected to music. The connections were endless. Nothing existed by itself.

From that day on I decided to live my life connecting everything—connecting the dots that made the full picture. I knew I wanted to be an actress, even at that age, and I realized that every single thing I did would now connect to my becoming an actress. Every person I met, every feeling I felt, would ultimately relate back to my future. I knew there wasn't anything that lived in isolation. (I've never heard anyone use the word score like that since, but that's not important.) The important thing was that from that day on, there wasn't anything that existed in and of itself. This was such an intense thought for an eight-year-old. I remember carrying it around with me and feeling as if I had really found the key to life. And if I could just continue to connect things, then everything would make a fuller picture for me than it already had.

Health is not just about weight or appearance, but rather a much bigger picture. I really believe that you can't be a healthy person unless everything is working together. True health comes only when every aspect of your life is integrated. Your body, your mind, your living space. Spend 30 days with me and you'll get more than an eating plan. I'll tell you not only what to eat and how to cook it, but also things to think about and tasks to do. You'll not only discover food to eat, but food for thought. Live in my world for 30 days and I know you will feel better. (At the very least, I guarantee you'll have a more organized house!) Together we're going to connect all kinds of dots.

God bless the World Wide Web! Ever since I created my website, ***www.Marilu.com,*** I've been able to create and customize this 30-day plan according to what you've asked for. Three out of four letters that I received asked me for more recipes, a typical meal plan, information regarding what I eat on an average day, and/or a 30-day menu that you can eat and still feed your kids.

I've been able to get a pretty good idea of who you are out there and, through that communication, what it is you're looking for. In general, you're busy and you want answers. You're usually caring for a family, but that doesn't mean you don't want to take care of yourself as well. You recognize that today we have a longer life expectancy, so we're seeking a better quality to our lives.

In *Total Health Makeover* I wanted to provide you with all of the information you would need to make some real changes in your life. Now that you have that information, you can't choose not to know anymore. You can't pretend you haven't been told about the evils of dairy, the benefits of food combining, or the difference between floaters and sinkers. This 30-day plan will make it easier for you to journey along a path of total health so it won't be so easy to make excuses. In this book, I'm giving you a map with 30 days of sample menus, easy-to-follow recipes, and all of the help you need to get and stay motivated. I'm even providing you with a list of things you'll need to complete our month together. I know you have questions. I've got your answers. And I swear to you, a lot of it is going to be FUN!

A friend called me recently and said, "Boy, I really have to go on your program. My two kids and my wife and I eat so poorly. We eat a lot of processed food. We eat a lot of junk food, a lot of fast food, but only my nine-year-old daughter is suffering. She's the only one with a weight problem."

I said to him, "Well, you know what? Your daughter's the natural healer. Her body knows that something is wrong. Her body is telling her she's not getting the right food. If you give her the right food, you won't believe how her body will respond."

That's how I felt about myself in the old days. I said to my friend, "I really hope you'll expose her to this program while she's nine years old so that she won't have to go through those painful teenage years, especially as her body changes."

If *I* had known when I was younger that I was a natural healer, I would have saved myself so much grief. I knew something was wrong. I knew that there was an answer out there. I just didn't know how to find it. Not knowing what to do combined with going on stupid diets and ruining my metabolism would haunt me for years to come far beyond my adolescence. But, for all of that grief, I'm glad that I went through what I went through (being overweight, having pimples and digestion problems), because it brought me to this place—a real sense of well-being, both mentally and physically. I was a natural healer, and my body knew that I was doing something that wasn't right. Through education and determination I've been able to turn my life around. And that's what it takes. Are you determined? Are you ready to make a change? I'm not telling you that you have to do *every* thing each of the thirty days. I'm simply asking you to try most of the suggestions and, more importantly, to *think* about your health in a way that maybe you haven't before. Remember, your health is not an isolated part of your life. I call my program the "Total Health Makeover" because it's about the total *you*.

Take the attitude that you're a work in progress. You're on this fantastic journey that's leading you down this road of health. It's not like you're on a diet when you follow my 30-day program—you're on a life path. It's one month out of your life; have fun with it and who knows—you might enjoy the process!

The 6 Most Frequently Asked Questions from *Total Health Makeover*

Before we get started, I would like to answer some of the more commonly asked questions you've had from *Total Health Makeover*. The following six questions are the ones most of you wrote about or asked me at book signings. (At least you know I read my e-mail!) Anyway, the first question has been the bane of my existence everywhere I go, so let's get this one out of the way up front!

1. "What the heck was that Turkey Tortilla Roll doing in the book?"

The number one question I've been asked since writing *Total Health Makeover* is about that damned turkey tortilla wrap! Let me say once and for all, for anybody reading this book, if you haven't read the first one, and you see that turkey tortilla wrap, the apple chutney at the bottom was supposed to be *beans!* This would have made it a good combination by making the tortilla and the turkey a complete protein. Also, that particular recipe was supposed to follow the meat chapter as an alternative in case some of you wanted to give up red meat and yet weren't ready to do food combining. Hopefully, this answers the thousands and thousands of you who called me on this one—good catch!

2. Where does tofu fit in when food combining?

A lot of you were confused about tofu because you didn't know that it is made from soybeans, which makes it a legume. And because it's a legume it is half starch, half protein. When you combine it with a starch it makes a full protein because the tofu has the amino acids that the starch is missing. Eating a legume with a meal that has both a starch and a protein will turn the starch part of the dish into a whole protein, thus making your entire meal a protein meal. A good example of this would be eating sushi. I love sushi, but without eating some type of legume it would be taboo for me. So I always order edamame (steamed soybeans) and eat them whenever I eat sushi to make the meal a complete protein.

3. What do you do if you hit a plateau?

Sometimes when dieting, your body will hit a plateau or a weight that you can't seem to break through. This can happen for any number of reasons. Your body could be rebelling at first from the changes you've made. Maybe you're eating too little and you've set yourself up for a famine by not eating enough. Your body may actually be hoarding the reserves and not burning the excess fat and calories. Or, you're eating too much overall or at one time. Your portions may have unknowingly increased because you've given up one thing and replaced it with too much of something else. Or, you could still be doing what I call the "Mommy Syndrome." (That's when you eat all the extra food off of everyone else's plate. You pick a little here and a little there, totally unaware of the extra portions.)

Maybe you're not exercising enough or you're not getting enough sleep. Both can affect weight loss. The best way to figure out the reason is to track what you eat and your activities by writing the information down in a notebook or journal.

It may be as simple as a lack of patience. Don't make yourself nuts. Give your body enough time to start seeing results. Your stress level can affect your weight loss as well. If you're stressed out, your body might have a tendency to hold on to everything inside. Even your breathing is affected. You might feel a little claustrophobic. Pay attention to what's happening around you when wondering why your weight loss has stalled.

To break this cycle, you might want to "shock" your system by doing something out of your regular routine. Whether it's eating smaller meals more frequently or stepping up the intensity of your workouts, you might want to try doing something a little different. Take a vacation from your usual schedule. I'm not saying you should go out and eat everything in sight or stop eating altogether. Just mix up your regime a little. I remember being in Las Vegas doing a movie once and I just felt that something wasn't working right in my body. So I stopped working out for a week and then started again with a lot of gusto. It was amazing how everything started to work again. I liken it to cleaning the heads of a cassette deck. Every now and then you have to wipe the slate clean to get maximum performance.

4. Can children eat on this program?

Children will benefit tremendously from not eating sugar and dairy and extra fat. My kids have eaten this way all of their lives and they are strong, healthy boys who very rarely get sick (knock wood). My children, of course, don't always food combine, but one thing I will tell you is my kids never have fruit juice after a meal because it gives them a sour stomach.

Something that I read while feeding my children early on was that children should not be given grains until they have teeth. (This makes so much sense!) It stands to reason that the development of teeth corresponds with the ability to digest grains. That's why we have canines to break the grains and molars to grind. Even if one tooth is in, it means that a child's stomach enzymes are now ready to break down the composition of the grains. Many people tend to give their babies grains too early; this causes discomfort in the child's tummy, making them gassy. If you have an infant who has been having these types of reactions after eating, try taking them off grains until they have a tooth and see if this doesn't solve your problem.

5. How do you get your spouse to join in?

I'm happy to say that this is not just a "chick" book. I've had so many guys on this program who have been thrilled by the results. Health is not gender biased. And in that same theory, neither is this 30-day program.

Marilu:

I heard you on the radio and you inspired me to try your program. I started eating fruit only in the morning, eliminated dairy, and started to properly food combine. In only a few weeks, I had lost seven pounds and my cholesterol dropped from 254 to 174. My doctor couldn't stop talking about my progress.

It has now been 3½ months, and I have lost 22 pounds, my skin has cleared up, a shoulder pain I had for two years is gone, and it's been almost effort free.

One of the nicest benefits of not buying all of that processed food and beverages is that I have saved so much money! Even spending more on organic food and fresh fruits doesn't come close to what I spent before just on diet soda and coffee! Do I sound excited about my health or what? Thanks!

Patrick Keeler

The important thing to remember on this program is that you have to do it for yourself. You really shouldn't use anyone else as the reason for getting healthy because more often than not you won't stay with it. When people ask me about encouraging others to get on this program before they themselves have tried it, I always think about what they tell you to do on an airplane during the safety announcement. In the event of an emergency, the flight attendant instructs you to put on your oxygen mask first so that you'll be able to help others around you. And that's my point about this program too. Don't worry about your spouse—yet. Take care of yourself first.

Hopefully the new streamlining in your life and body, the empowerment you'll feel from your commitment, and the energy that you'll now have to put toward your work and relationships will be contagious. Discover a life filled with vibrant and exuberant health and I'll bet everyone around you will say, "I want to do what you're doing!"

6. Do I ever cheat?

The answer is YES! I actually encourage cheating. If you don't cheat *once in a while*, you can't test your progress. You just can't. If I hadn't had a wild gelati night, and then stood over a toilet bowl all night thereafter, I would never have appreciated how good it feels to have given up dairy once and for all. You have to check your progress once in a while, and you can do it by cheating. There are some steps I would never cheat on and some steps I cheat on once in a while.

It's impossible to eat a 100 percent chemical-free diet. I eat in restaurants, I eat on airplanes, and sometimes when I can't find a fruit-sweetened ketchup, I'll eat regular ketchup and stuff like that. But at the very least, I do not have processed chemical–laden foods in my house. And I would say probably 80 to 85 percent of the time everything I eat is chemical free. But I don't live in a vacuum. I think that's impossible. When discovering and developing this program, I wanted to find something that I could live with in the real world. That was my main objective in finding a program that worked for me. I didn't want to feel as though in order to look my best I had to go off somewhere and create this person and then be her only for the weekend. I wanted to be a healthy human being able to exist among people and to be social too.

I never drink coffee or smoke. If there's a little bit of caffeine in a piece of nondairy sugar-free chocolate that I might have the night before my period, it doesn't stop me from eating it, but otherwise I don't drink caffeinated sodas or decaffeinated coffee.

About twice a year, I'll have a dessert that has refined sugar in it. I do, however, eat desserts sweetened with raw honey, barley malt, maple syrup, rice syrup, unrefined sugar, or fruit. I *never* eat red meat or anything made with a beef stock. I never eat chicken, but my boys do. I personally find it too strong a protein for females, but I get plenty of protein from fish and bean products (especially soy).

I avoid dairy completely but I'm sure that that sugary dessert I eat every now and then might have a little milk in it. I never eat cheese, though. In fact, I haven't eaten cheese since 1982.

In terms of cheating on fat, it would only be eating *more* of the same foods that I usually do. It's a volume issue for me. Sometimes I might eat other foods that are higher in fat. For example, I love these dairy-free, sugar-free doughnuts that pack 20 grams of fat. They're not part of my steady diet, but occasionally I can't resist. But, for the most part, I eat low-fat meals. By virtue of your following this program you will be doing the same thing.

There are days when I don't food combine. Maybe I'm exhausted, and all day long I have that mindless, stupid, hungry, tired feeling that makes you eat without thinking. Afterwards, however, I find myself feeling uncomfortable. I probably food combine perfectly only 75 percent of the time. I know I can fix practically any bad combination by eating some cooked soybeans, which I always have in my refrigerator. I'm always aware of how I feel when I don't properly combine what I eat, and that's an important part of the process. Having an awareness of what you eat and how certain foods affect your body both physically and mentally is a big part of gaining control over your health and well-being.

Although I exercise regularly, I'm not getting the same amount of exercise that I was getting when I was doing *Chicago* on Broadway, but my weight is the same. No matter what, I make it a point to break a sweat every day, even if it's only for ten minutes.

Sleep is still my biggest problem. I'm just not a sleeper. I'm lucky I don't need a lot. But sometimes I don't even get what I need. It just depends on what else is going on in my life.

Of all of the ten steps, I definitely believe that gusto is the most important. I can't think of one interview this past year where I didn't have gusto. (It's easy to have gusto when you love what you're doing!) Gusto is really being in the moment. Without it everything seems a little off. Your whole being screams discomfort and the body language you reflect makes you look even worse. But don't forget that gusto can also mean having downtime and enjoying being by yourself.

I hope this answers your most frequently asked questions from *Total Health Makeover*. (I can't wait to hear your new ones from this book!)

1

What to Expect from Each Week

Aside from complete food plans for thirty days, each day also consists of seven tips. There's a Motivational Tip, Exercise Tip, Food Tip, Organizational Tip, Beauty Tip, Spa on a Budget Tip (a.k.a. more bang for your buck!), and even a Total Health Fakeover Tip. I'm not asking you to do each tip every day, but try to read them and accomplish as many as you can. For example, if a particular tip tells you to buy a certain kind of shampoo, you don't *have* to buy it that day. I'm just suggesting that the next time you're buying shampoo to keep it in mind. Another reason for all of the tips is to get you thinking about something other than food. When those impossible cravings happen, you can channel that energy into organizing your closet, counter, or kitchen. Whatever. Next time you're on the phone, tackle that junk drawer. Instead of mindlessly sitting in front of the television set, give yourself a facial or do some sit-ups during the commercials. You found that extra time to eat—you can find that extra time to organize. All of these daily tips can be tackled in small increments.

Who knows, maybe six months from now you might say to yourself, "You know what? I remember Marilu told me to organize my sock drawer. I think I'll do that." Or, you might remember one of my Total Health Fakeover tips when you have to be somewhere and aren't quite feeling up to the task. The idea is to have some fun and learn new things that you may never have tried before. But *please*, don't get overwhelmed. These are all things that I do in my life, but I certainly don't do *all* of them at one time. I just want to get you into a mode where you take a look at your life and see all the areas you might want to improve. I know that you're busy (we all are), and you don't have a lot of free time (none of us do). But don't you agree that things are easier when your life is more organized and working like a well-oiled machine? Besides, once you take the time to organize something well, who knows—you might be inspired to keep it that way. Think of each day like you are back in school and the tips are fun homework assignments that'll benefit you. If you can't get them all done, that's fine, because luckily, you're not being graded—you're being *upgraded*.

This 30-day program has been divided into five sections. Countdown, Purple Week (a.k.a. "Boot Camp"), Blue Week, Green Week, and Yellow Week.

Countdown (Or, How to Avoid the Last Supper—or Two)

The first four days of this program begin with what I refer to as "Countdown." For those of you who have not already implemented some of the original ten steps from *Total Health Makeover*, Countdown is four days where you're going to prepare yourself and your body for the rest of the program. Countdown was created for all those people (you know who you are) who like to go on a wild binge prior to starting a new diet. It would be great if you could have the proper mindset from the start of this program that this is not an end, but a beginning. A really common mistake people make prior to starting any weight loss program is they use their new beginning as an excuse to go crazy and overindulge themselves right before they get started. Sometimes they keep doing it and they never actually *get* started. A few years ago, two of my sisters and I went to a health spa. One of my sisters showed up in Los Angeles on Friday afternoon, and by the time we left for the spa on Sunday, she had eaten her way through L.A., gaining five pounds in the process. It took until Wednesday just to catch up to where she was before she came to town! This is the reason I've put Countdown into the program. I don't want you to have to spend the first four days of Boot Camp catching up. It's like starting with a clean slate. Who wants to spend all of his or her time undoing the damage? Countdown is so you can avoid the "Last Supper" and get the most out of Boot Camp. The idea of Countdown is not to go crazy but to become aware of how you feel and the effect certain foods (or lack of certain foods) are having on your body. It's like a mental and physical preparation. Think of it as the buffer between your old habits and your new life.

I made such a big deal out of doing one step at a time in *Total Health Makeover*, and I still believe, for this program to be its most effective, you ought to experience each step one by one. But the bottom line is this: you won't hurt yourself by going on this program, no matter where you're starting from. You might be the picture of health already, so you're just going to feel even better. Conversely, you may be so far away from the animal you were meant to be that you're going to see dramatic results. And let's just say no matter what steps you did from *Total Health Makeover*, I'm asking you to live your first four days with **NO RED MEAT, NO SUGAR, NO DAIRY PRODUCTS, AND NO ALCOHOL**. (The last of which isn't one of the ten steps, but avoiding it should be part of any cleansing period.) If you're already dairy free or sugar free, that's a great start. If you're all four, then you can skip Countdown and proceed straight to Boot Camp. I picked four days for Countdown because if all of this is new to you, that's how long it takes to get some of the physical cravings out of your system. For this program, I'm not going to be a maniac about your giving up caffeine, because I know that a lot of you will never give up coffee and that's fine . . . for now. (You can use soy or rice milk in your coffee instead of cow's milk.)

Countdown is also the time that I want you to get acquainted with the big picture of the next 30 days. Countdown is like getting ready to leave on a fabulous 30-day trip, but *this* trip is the trip of *your life!* Before you pack you have to gather everything you'll need for that journey, right? It's the same with this program. It's like reading the directions to a new board game you've never played.

I'm not asking you to change everything about your way of life during Countdown. It's just a good way of preparing yourself for the rest of the program. I just want you to

3

see how much meat, dairy, alcohol, and sugar affect your body. Additionally, if you do go through any sort of healing crises during the first four days, I want you to understand that it's from the foods you've eliminated from your diet rather than from this program.

Understanding the Personality of Each Week

Each week on this program has been given a color that corresponds to its level of difficulty and to my infamous "Rainbow Theory." Anyone who knows me has without a doubt heard my Rainbow Theory *at least* once. It's my consummate description of what most of us go through in our lives, so I thought it was befitting to label each week of the plan accordingly.

I realized that there had to be a way to describe the cycle I was continually finding myself going through in my quest to lose weight and get fit prior to adapting my current way of life. One day, I linked into this idea that all of the colors in a rainbow correlated perfectly to that vicious cycle.

Try and picture in your mind a rainbow. In my theory, each of the colors represents a different period and behavioral pattern in your life. You wake up one morning and you say to yourself, "That's it! Today I am starting my new fitness program and this time, *nothing* can stop me!" You are in the Purple phase (which is also the color of the first week on this 30-day program). When you're in Purple, your attitude is come hell or high water, you're going to stick to a program with pure perfection. It's cattle prodder to the brain time. You're going to eat perfectly, exercise religiously, and organize strategically. And then one day you wake up and realize you're starting to feel really good about your progress, and it might be okay to get out there again. You're moving into the Blue phase (week two on the program). As humans, we are inherently social animals, and besides, you're feeling so good about your success in Purple, you want to show off a bit in Blue. You might be a little nervous because you haven't been disciplined long enough to feel that the program is really part of you, but one day you wake up and everything in your life is in its place. You're feeling perfectly balanced and you have entered the often-strived-for phase of Green (week three of the program). People who are in Green exercise regularly and can socialize without slipping up too much and still feel really good about themselves. Usually this phase doesn't last very long because it's very hard to exist in the center. You wake up one day and realize that your Green is turning to Yellow (week four of the program), which really means that you're now integrating this program into your everyday life, but you are not doing everything 100 percent of the time. In real life, your pendulum is always swinging even if the swings aren't extreme. I wanted to show you in this program how to be a little wilder than center (bigger meals, social drinking, desserts, snacks, etc.) and yet still stay within the guidelines of this plan with relative ease. You'll be bending the rules but without having to pay a huge price. Beyond Yellow are two colors that I did not include in my plan because they're too far away from where we should be aiming—the worlds of Orange and Red. Orange is when your social life has started to consume any and all focus you once had on your physical well-being. You haven't been to the gym in weeks, and you're so bloated from eating and drinking that even your black jeans make you look fat! You're a total party animal, booking lunches, dinners, and happy-hour buffets. And Red! Well, in Red, you're either lying on the floor with drool coming out of your mouth, or . . . you're in Italy (my favorite place to be in Red!). After you finish the program, hopefully, you will become more disciplined about your habits and can avoid slipping into the worlds of Orange and Red. But even if you occasionally feel like your pendulum is starting to swing way out of balance, you may want to go back to the week of Blue or Purple to recapture that sense of order. Ideally, you will fluctuate between Green and Yellow all of the time. But, there *will* be times that you'll fall off the plan (like vacations or times of stress). Know that you can get back on track.

Once you experience the four colors of this plan, you'll have a better sense of which color best fits your needs. For example, maybe the discipline of "Purple Week" is working really well for you. You might consider staying in Purple for several weeks until you feel you're ready to move on to Blue. The key is to be in touch with your body and how you're feeling in each phase so that you can recognize what you need to become your B.E.S.T.

Purple Week, a.k.a. "Boot Camp"

Boot Camp, which is the first five days with menus of this program, is another name for Purple week. (Notice, it's only 5 days instead of 7. Yea!) Boot Camp will be a lot easier to get through if you've already gone through four days of Countdown. It won't seem so dramatic to someone who's already experienced how much better he or she feels by eliminating those four health robbers (sugar, meat, dairy, alcohol) right from the start. To some of you, however, Boot Camp may feel like a really strict diet. That's the purpose of going through Boot Camp. I am going to ask you to adhere to the rules *during the first nine days* of this program (the four days of Countdown and the five days of Boot Camp). In fact, think of it like a game. It works like this: if you break any of the food rules in those first nine days, you should go back to the beginning of the program and start all over. Really make a commitment to yourself to get through the first nine days of this plan without falling off. It's an important time because you will teach yourself how to taste flavors in food again. You will be retraining your palate. Maybe you'll be trying some new foods or some tips that you've never tried before. Open yourself up to the experience and the liberation of all of these new ideas.

Blue Week, Green Week, Yellow Week

As you progress into Blue week, you will see that I gradually start to introduce more complex ingredients, though the recipes remain simple and easy to prepare. Green week allows you to start having rewards in terms of snacks and desserts, and Yellow week takes you to the end of the 30-day cycle where we bend the rules a little and include a celebration dinner.

You won't feel deprived in terms of how much food you're going to eat on my program because the portions are rather generous. However, I am not in your body, so the portions are suggestions and should be adjusted accordingly. But as I always say—if you improve the quality of the food you eat, the quantity takes care of itself. The recipes contained in this book are really tasty and delicious. The bottom line is simple. If you follow each week's plan, by the end of the 30 days, you will look and feel better.

Your body will be experiencing so many changes as you start this program. Some are quite noticeable and others more subtle. Many of you don't realize that feeling healthy is an elusive thing, albeit very attainable. It's defined so differently for different people. You're going to have a better sense of well-being. You'll see that your highs and lows are no longer from a synthetic source, like sugar. You'll more than likely feel a steadier stream of energy. You'll be tired at night and better able to sleep. This program has been designed to change your knowledge and the way you view your health and food. As you become more aware of what you are consuming, you inevitably become more conscious of your choices. You'll start to taste flavors that were always there but no longer hidden under a layer of butter. Once you start to taste real food, your cravings for the fake stuff will be alleviated or will go away completely.

You'll have cleaner breath and cleaner breathing on this plan too. (There's nothing worse than fermented breath from eating sugar and dairy products.) And once you're off dairy, you will notice an obvious difference in the amount of mucus in your throat and nose. There's going to be less dependency on chemical objects outside yourself as well. Your energy will feel more constant instead of those artificially induced peaks and valleys.

I designed this 30-day program with its meal plan and seven tips so that every day there's something different. The tips are meant to give you ideas. Something on these pages is going to spark your imagination, and maybe you'll accomplish all of them one day. But don't be hard on yourself, and don't be so maniacal or so obsessed that you're losing sight of what we're trying to do here, and that is to make our lives streamlined and easier to deal with. You know, what we're trying to create here is a well-oiled machine where everything seems organic and so much a part of us that it's as natural as brushing our teeth. I don't want you to think "She's asking me to do seven things before I even have my breakfast!" What have you got to lose except some weight, some old ideas, and some old health problems?

Don't think of me as someone who's dragging you kicking and screaming to your health. You shouldn't think of this as deprivation. It's not a sentence.

Think of me instead as someone who is trying to put you into a winning syndrome mode. Instead of taking out our frustrations on our bodies, I'm saying take it out on your closet or your sock drawer. Shift the energy. See your life in a new way. Think of it like this. Pretend you're looking through the lens of a camera. This is the lens through which you view your life, your habits, and everything else that influences your health and well-being. On this 30-day journey, I'm asking you to slightly shift the angle of that lens. See the same things from a new perspective. Look at your living space, your clothes, the way you apply your makeup, stock your refrigerator, the way your body looks, etc. . . . (Remember . . . everything is connected to everything.) Hopefully, by turning that lens in a new direction, the focus is going to be sharper and clearer. It may be different from anything you've ever done before, maybe a little quirkier or even radical. But experience this for thirty days and have fun with it. For 30 days, I'm asking you to live in my world. Take that ride with me. Now, you can laugh and say, "This girl is so out there. No wonder she acts like she does on David Letterman!" But, it's worth a shot if I can help get you on that road to better health, energy, stamina, and well-being.

Why I've Chosen the Foods I've Chosen

If you're wondering why you're going to be eating certain foods on this diet, the following list of vitamins and minerals will explain why I've chosen the foods I've chosen.

Vitamin	Key Facts	Sources
A	Listed as beta-carotene; improves weak eyesight; builds resistance to respiratory infections; promotes healthy hair, skin, teeth, and gums	Leafy green vegetables, carrots, sweet potatoes, winter squash, cantaloupe
B-1	Must be replaced daily; promotes normal appetite, fights car-, air-, and sea-sickness; improves mental attitude	Whole grains, oatmeal, legumes, bran, dried yeast

B-2	Known as riboflavin; helps eliminate sore mouth, lips, and tongue; alleviates eye fatigue	Leafy green vegetables, fish
B-6	Must be present for antibody and red blood cell production; helps prevent skin disorders; alleviates nausea; reduces leg cramps	Fish, shellfish, wheat bran, wheat germ, cantaloupe, cabbage, blackstrap molasses
B-12	Promotes growth and increases appetite; improves concentration, memory, and balance; prevents anemia; decreases irritability	Fish, shellfish, eggs
C	Essential for formation of collagen, the primary constituent of bone, cartilage, and connective tissue; destroyed by carbon monoxide; alleviates prickly heat; acts as a natural laxative; decreases blood cholesterol	Citrus fruits, strawberries, green and leafy vegetables, cantaloupe, green pepper, cauliflower, potatoes, sweet potatoes
D	Acquired through sunlight or diet; promotes strong bones and teeth; helps prevent colds when taken with vitamins A and C	Sardines, salmon, tuna, egg yolk
E	An active antioxidant; destroyed by heat and freezing temperatures; alleviates fatigue; prevents scar formation; prevents cell membrane damage; speeds the healing of burns	Wheat germ, vegetable oils, broccoli, brussels sprouts, whole-grain cereals, spinach, soybeans

How to Get Past the Difficult Parts

If you let this program become a game, you'll end up having an easier time by not allowing yourself to become frustrated and self-defeating, especially if you're not seeing results right away. Say to yourself, "Hey, let me just try some of this stuff on for size and see how it works."

Years ago when I was involved with someone in Alcoholics Anonymous, I got the literature for Al-Anon, and something they recommended (actually a lot of things they recommended) really worked. They said that if you're helping someone stay sober it is best to have them avoid being H.A.L.T.—hungry, angry, lonely, tired. For *this* 30-day program I have changed this acronym to S.A.L.T.: *starving*, angry, lonely, tired. I think a *little* bit of hunger is not a bad thing because you want to wake up and say, "Ooh, I'm really looking forward to that breakfast," or "Wow, let's go out for a really great dinner." But don't ever let yourself get to the point of *starving*. I think that's one of the biggest problems with so-called dieting. Sometimes you get past the point of hunger and you're so famished that all want to do is stuff your face. You don't allow twenty minutes to go by so that it sinks into your brain that you've now put something in your stomach. You can't get food in there fast enough. It's not even food anymore—it's gut fill.

I'm not looking for you to be starving on this program. That's the worst thing that you could do. (All right, Boot Camp may be a little less food than you'll eventually get.) But, if what I'm recommending is not enough food for you (I doubt it overall), then eat a little more. If it's too much at one time, then save some of it and eat it later. I want you to get used to eating about every three hours so that you are constantly stoking your internal furnace. I just keep getting an image of all these little guys at work in your belly. It's like you're an ocean liner (think *QE2* please, not the *Titanic*). In order to keep your engines at full steam ahead, you've got to keep shoveling in that coal. You've got to keep those furnaces burning so that the ship is running at its optimum.

As I keep telling you, one of the biggest reasons people don't lose weight is that they don't eat enough. On my program, even *during* Boot Camp you're not going to be starving yourself. You're just going to be eating in proper combination. You're not going to be eating the foods that take energy from you. And you're going to be eating enough of it at each meal to feel satisfied. So the "S" for starving is the worst thing. You can't let that happen.

A lot of people wrote to me and said that they couldn't go the whole morning just eating fruit. A lot of you said you're getting up at six o'clock and then not eating until one o'clock at lunch. That's not good. You can't spend all of that time trying to work without something substantial in your stomach. But the wrong food in the morning will make you tired. You should always feel energized by the foods you eat. That's why on this program I'm giving you fruit in the morning to kick start your system and to set up your stomach enzymatically, and two hours later (or less, if necessary) you will be eating whole grain toast, cereal, or an egg white omelet, etc., to give you energy until lunch. If your body is moving and working efficiently, you're going to need food. And you might get a little hungry, but remember, you're not allowed to feel like you're starving.

When you're *angry*, you're emotionally upset. Maybe somebody disappointed you, or maybe you disappointed yourself. Whatever the reasons, we've all got the same old "comfort food" trigger. It's like when you fell down as a child and your mother instantly said, "Oh, honey, you fell and hurt yourself. Here, have a cookie." From that moment on, we've all been trained to associate eating something with feeling better. Usually the thing we ate was something bad for us that was supposed to make us feel better, but all it did, really, was overpower what we just experienced by creating a whole new set of problems or emotions.

It's understandable that a lot of our feelings of anger or frustration go into our eating habits. Even to this day, I'll have a bad conversation with someone, and I'll find myself standing at the refrigerator. I'll think to myself, what am I doing? Even though the food in my refrigerator is good, and I really can't get into trouble eating it, it's still a conditioned response that somebody made me feel bad, or something made me feel frustrated, so I feel like I want to eat whether or not I'm hungry. And usually, I want to eat something crunchy and salty, because it's noisy and aggressive, or I want to eat something sweet and creamy because it's comforting and soothing. We put so many of our feelings under that

11

anger umbrella. All it makes us want to do is act out in some way, so we take it out on our bodies. If you want to grab something left over from your lunch, then fine. But we still shouldn't be acting out with food, even if it's good food. We women, especially, tend to do this. We're so afraid of our angry feelings. We hide, we mask, we soothe, and we "put out" so much to other people that we feel we have the right to "take in" food.

Lonely can be construed two ways. Most mothers out there would love that lonely feeling once in a while. Lonely sometimes sounds really good. If anything, you'd like to use your lonely feelings to maybe throw a party for one, take a hot bath (uninterrupted), and order great room service in a fabulous hotel. But, that's not loneliness. That's being alone with yourself.

I'm talking about feeling real loneliness. It's always cooking for one when you don't have enough going on in your life, or you wish you were responsible for somebody else. You can also live with a house full of people and *still* feel lonely and misunderstood. Or you can feel lonely because you're with people all the time, and they can eat what they want and you don't understand why you can't.

Whatever the reasons, you can feel lonely because you're simply not connected to your body or to other people. We're all looking to feel like we're part of something. We're looking to have our minds and our bodies and our health and everything else we do conveniently accessible in one package and to feel interconnected. Before I figured out all of this, I knew that there was this healthy, thin, happy, energetic girl living inside of me. I'd seen glimpses of her. I'd seen childhood snapshots of her. And it was only an issue of rediscovering those emotions that brought me to where I am today. My physical world really had to catch up with my mental perception, because no matter how much gusto I had, I would look in the mirror and know that something was not right at 174 pounds.

You have to remember to always remain a work in progress. If we're lucky enough and smart enough, we're always going to remain students of life. I'm always learning new things. I'm always trying to figure things out. When you stop questioning and learning, you're dead—either emotionally or physically.

And that brings me to the "T" in SALT—*tired*. I would go so far as to say that 90 percent of our exhaustion is from not eating well and a lack of energy. It's food-induced, and it's habit-induced. And I think that so much of that is going to go away once you get rolling on this 30-day plan. If there has to be one consistent thing I've heard from people who have been on this program, it's that they have more energy. Most of your tiredness is going to be alleviated, but remember—we still get tired. People are still parents who have sick children, career people who are up all night, or have careers *and* families. There are going to be those times in your life when you are going to feel exhausted. It's during those times that you have to be especially careful of the kind of food that you put into your mouth. Those are the times that I think are the real danger zones that become difficult on any kind of program. I don't care what kind of eater you are, you have to watch for those land mines. There are those times when we end up giving in to whatever is available rather than finding whatever is good for us. You have to learn to flex your discipline muscle (more about that later). You have to really practice. Also, if you surround yourself with better food, even if you do grab something, at least it's not junk. Just become aware of *why* you're grabbing it. You've either put yourself in a state of deprivation (Starving), or emotional upheaval (Angry), or disconnection (Lonely), or exhaustion (Tired). And it's those four areas that are always very difficult to chart a course. You have to be really careful because that's where anything can fall apart, not just your eating habits.

Setting Up Your Program Journal

In *Total Health Makeover*, I talked at length about setting up a journal to help track your daily progress. What I suggest is getting a spiral notebook and numbering each page to correspond with the corresponding day of the program. (You'll do this during Countdown.)

Check off all of your program activities for the day. Include any exercise, tips you did, number of hours of sleep from the night before, and a complete list of everything you eat and drink. Keep it simple, but be sure you make your entries daily. It's still the best way to keep track of your progress along the way.

13

One final suggestion as you get started on your 30-day plan. Take some before and after photos of yourself. Take the photos from all angles so that you can really see every side of your body. Do them from the front, each side, and from behind. Take a close-up and a full body shot. This step is completely optional, but you will most certainly see a difference, especially in your face, after thirty days. You know the old saying—every picture tells a story!

2

Evaluating Your Assets and Liabilities

NEWS FLASH: No matter what we do, we're not going to be Cindy Crawford. Cindy Crawford is a genetically near-perfect specimen of a human being. We can go on every diet in the world, but it still might not turn us into a supermodel. (Even supermodels have to work at being healthy.) But that's all right, because this program is designed to help *you* become the B.E.S.T. version of yourself.

Before you start this program it's a good idea to get a complete physical so that you can monitor your progress over time. Measure your height and weight and take a series of blood tests that evaluate your cholesterol, your LDL and HDL ratio, your glucose, blood type, and blood pressure, etc. You should really have this done at least once a year anyway.

Evaluating Your Assets and Liabilities

Ask anyone what his or her best and worst physical features are, and no doubt you'll get a very strong response. I tested this theory by asking my family and friends this question, and every single one of them had an answer. They knew their bodies well enough to know what they like to show and what they like to cover up. What surprised me the most was that in some cases, they knew exactly what to do and in other cases they were completely clueless. Some people accentuated things that were not their assets but rather, their liabilities, while others knew exactly how to show off their best "stuff."

What are your assets and liabilities? Take a good look at your body and acknowledge what they are. Look at your body in terms of the pluses and minuses. Instead of looking at yourself and seeing only the negative, look at yourself and see all the great things that you have. Know that after thirty days, your assets are just going to get that much better, and your liabilities are going to change, too. I always know that when I go into Purple mode, my good gets better before my bad does. It works in reverse too. If I pig out, my problem areas will get hit hardest first. For example, I know that my stomach is the area on my body that I like the least and my legs are the best part. No matter what I weighed over the years, whenever I started putting a little energy into eating well and exercising daily, the first thing to respond was always my legs. Prior to *this* program I never stayed on anything long enough to see any response in my stomach area, but it has always been the first thing to thicken if I spend two or three days abusing myself! My jeans get too tight and I get this spare tire feeling as well as little haunches on my lower back. The point is that you have to stay with something long enough for all of your parts to improve. Fake yourself out for a while until they do by becoming a masterful camouflage dresser. Wear clothes that hide the liabilities until they too become assets. Or like my friend Caroline Aaron says, "If you can't hide it, decorate it." I'm not suggesting that you run out and get horizontal-striped stretch pants or anything like that. I'm saying celebrate the good parts and embrace the bad ones until they get good. They *will* change because everything's going to improve.

Looking at Your Body from a Different Angle

When most people look at themselves in a mirror they look straight on and evaluate themselves only from the front. If you were to look at your body sideways in a mirror, and I mean *really* look at your body sideways and pretend that there's this imaginary line down the middle of your body what would you see reflected back? Would you see an erect and totally balanced body or would you see one with rounded shoulders and a potbelly? There's a saying I learned from studying macrobiotics that goes like this: "The bigger the front, the bigger the back." That means that on either side of that imaginary line, the two sides are equal. That's why you'll rarely see somebody with slumped shoulders who doesn't have a potbelly. You never see somebody with splayed legs who doesn't have saddlebags coming out. You'll notice that if your posture gets better, it'll appear as if you've already lost five pounds.

Think of your abdomen as the center of your body. Everything within our bodies stems from this center. It's not a coincidence that the center of a woman is where babies come from. It's a life-giving force. If we're uptight, we hold tension in our center. We hold anger in our center and almost every other emotion, positive and negative. As a dancer, I was always taught to find my center in order to have perfect balance. Without your center, you have nothing that supports the rest of your body.

Creating an awareness of your center starts with proper digestion. It's getting in touch with your inner self. If you are having digestion problems, a distended stomach from a spastic colon, or an inflamed bowel, you will be out of balance in your center.

Women are especially prone to feeling out of balance because we get our periods every month. We feel bloated and fat, and we just accept that this is part of our lives. But, once we get our periods, that bloaty feeling dissipates, and we feel better, taller, thinner, and healthier, right? We can feel that way all of the time.

Finding your center is also about improving your posture and allowing every movement to stem from that point. (You want to feel like your belly button is up against the wall of your back.) It makes complete sense that if your center is off kilter, the rest of your body will be too. A lot of people can't find their center because their digestion is off, and they keep doing stomach crunches, and that's simply not the answer. You can do all the sit-ups in the world, but if you have an inflamed bowel, there's no way that you're ever going to have a flat stomach. A protruding stomach has more to do with your whole digestive system. Remember, humans have 27 feet of intestines. A lot stems from what you're putting into your body. If you don't respect the quality of the food you eat, it's like using flimsy cheap materials that lack quality to build your home. Eventually, your house will become dilapidated and fall apart. On this program, as your digestion improves, you will begin to straighten out your body and start standing more upright. Your stomach is definitely going to get flatter and your body is going to adjust itself by lifting and bringing everything more to your center. In order to flatten your stomach, you don't just work on your stomach—you work on your digestion and you strengthen your back as well. The back supports the stomach. (Remember, everything is connected to everything.)

Think of your stomach as this "work center." If it's not in balance, your whole body will be out of whack. Have you ever noticed that you can overeat one night, and when you wake up the next morning you say, "Oh, I feel fine, maybe a little bloated but I still look thin everywhere else, so no harm done"? And you can overeat again the next day and still squeak by. But after the third time, it's like the little cells in your stomach scream, "Disperse!" Suddenly, it seems like all that excess fat floods all over your body. You wake up after that third day and say, "I'm so fat." You might have been getting away with it on the scale but after that third day—watch out!

As you check your progress from week to week, you're not going to believe how things are going to start adjusting around that center. Finding your center is an integral part in the success of this 30-day program. You can practice balancing your center anywhere, anytime. When you're sitting in the car, check to see if you're slouching in the driver's seat or if you're sitting up really straight. Think of that imaginary center as running right down the core of your body, connecting your belly button to your back, pulling everything up, and helping everything adjust.

Your center is finding that imaginary line that divides your body in two from every angle. Once you get in touch with your center you won't believe how great it feels. Everything in your body starts to improve. It's like having the right wiring.

Your energy is better, your posture is better, the spring in your step is better, your results from exercise and especially your digestion just gets better and better! It's my goal that after the first nine days on this program (Countdown and Boot Camp), you'll tap in to find your center and start to not only recognize the difference but to also really enjoy the feeling. I want you to say, "Wow, my hard work is paying off!"

We've come to expect a pill to cure a headache, to cure indigestion, to cure PMS, and to hopefully one day cure cancer and AIDS. We're expecting this miracle whenever we swallow a pill. We endow this pill with tremendous power and we honor it. We respect it. We reach for it. We seek it. We put all of our faith in it. Think of the size of a pill. Can you imagine how much power there is in an entire plate of food? Do you realize how much power there is in the human mind? Have you any idea how much power there is in your attitude?

Depending on your perspective, it's limitless. Adjusting your attitude in any situation has the power to overwhelm you, satisfy you, or change your life. It's really the same thing with food. A plate of food has the power to overwhelm you, or it has the power to overjoy you. It can affect you physically, emotionally, or mentally. If you're in a good frame of mind, food is what it's supposed to be: life-giving, natural, and organic to your needs. If you're in a bad frame of mind, food can become a source of comfort or punishment. Avoiding self-sabotage in whatever area is the real trick to being successful.

Your Feet Are Your Foundation

If your stomach is your center then it makes sense that your feet are the foundation that keeps your body firmly planted. Like a skyscraper, without a solid foundation, your body would simply falter without the proper footing. Sometimes we need a little help. Like finding my center, discovering the benefits of orthotics (or shoe inserts) had a tremendous impact on improving my body. In 1984, after filming the movie *Perfect*, I was much heavier than I had been before I started. My body was way off, and I wasn't happy about it. The good news was that I was scheduled to go off to Spain to do another movie.

It was right before that trip to Spain that I discovered orthotics. I saw my personal trainer (back in the days when I had a personal trainer) just before I left, and he had me walk across the room. He noticed that I walked a little lopsided because I had one hip that was slightly higher than the other.

I also had such a high arch in my right foot that it was not really connecting with the ground. He put a lift in my left shoe and an arch in my right shoe, and he had me walk across the room again. I started to walk perfectly balanced with my hips the same level and my right foot in contact with the ground. With each step, I was determined to teach myself how to walk again from a new perspective.

When I arrived in Spain, I didn't have to film for the first ten days—so I decided I would put my best foot forward and lose those unwanted and unneeded pounds. It became a game for me to be by myself, keep a diary, and to start walking differently. I decided to retrain my whole body because I had felt completely out of balance. I figured if I wanted to correct the problem, I would have to start from scratch. I would have to reteach my body to do the simple things like stand and walk and even sit because even when I sat, I sat with my legs open and not parallel and I was starting to form saddlebags. Every time I sat in a chair I became conscious of keeping my feet, knees, and hips parallel. If I sat in a car—same thing. Everywhere I sat (even on the potty), I readjusted my position. What ended up happening was that I could feel my whole body realigning itself. It was as if my skeleton had straightened up! I had big hips before that trip, and afterwards, within eight weeks, I lost three inches! Once I got upright, straightened my posture, and made my feet straight, I realized that everything just started to get leaner because my pelvic structure and feet were no longer splayed. I completely changed my walk and my posture. I walked everywhere in Spain, and by the time I started filming I was already seeing an enormous improvement.

Orthotics

When I returned from Spain I saw a podiatrist, the fabulous Dr. Richard Rupp, who fitted me with custom-made orthotics. I don't know if every single person needs them, but what I do know is that every family member or friend of mine who has gotten them on my recommendation has significantly improved their body and/or their ability to walk or run. My husband Rob, in fact, was never able to run beyond a half a mile without suffering from groin and hip pain. Now he runs a 5K every day and a 10K on the weekends without any discomfort whatsoever because of orthotics. Maybe getting orthotics would help you too.

Think of your feet as the foundation that supports the rest of the "building" that is your body. There are 26 bones in each of your feet. At birth, your foot is almost devoid of bone and is made up of mostly cartilage tissue. The average arch does not become fully developed until we're around 18, and the foot itself not until around the age of 20! Your foot is very pliable, especially as a child. If you didn't properly take care of your feet as a child, chances are you're paying for it now as an adult. (I ruined my feet wearing a lot of stupid shoes as a teenager. I remember squeezing my size 7½ feet into a trendy pair of 6½'s that I just loved.) Your feet are the main support system for everything else. If you're out of balance when you walk, surely the rest of the body will suffer because it has to work overtime to compensate for the weakness in the structure. Dr. Timothy Liddy, D.P.M., who has a podiatric practice in West Hollywood, California, was interviewed for this book about the practical use of orthotics in everyday life. He explained to me that an orthotic is a specific functional device, available by prescription, to help create a functional balance between the foot and the body. An orthotic is different from an arch support in that an arch support simply fills the arch, and that can be made from foam or leather, like a Dr. Scholl's insert. Those can be useful because they serve to help keep the foot from overpronating so much. An orthotic is a prescription device, made by a doctor who is trained in biomechanics and making the devices.

In order to create a true orthotic, the doctor must have a thorough understanding of each individual's biomechanics. Biomechanics is the term used to describe the relationship between one joint to the next. How the foot functions relative to the ankle, the ankle relative to the knee, the knee relative to the hip, the hip relative to the lower back, and so on (just like the song). So when the doctor looks at someone's biomechanics, he or she assesses how they look when they're sitting, non-weight-bearing, or how they're standing, weight-bearing, and in gait, as they're walking. After reviewing each of these specific locations of the body, the doctor gets an idea of their posture.

Dr. Liddy says that he is really looking for the ranges of motion. And after reviewing thousands of people's ranges of motions, we've come to term what the normal limits of a range of motion of a particular joint should be. So when you start from the foot, you look at the big toe joint, and you look at the joints in the middle of the foot, and you look at the joints in the ankle, and then in the knee, and then in the hip. You evaluate each of these and determine how far off they are from what we term as normal.

The normal range of motion is best described when you take the perfect body and you classify it by where the muscles attach and how the joint optimally functions. That would be a perfect body. Now, very few of us have that. Maybe an elite athlete has exceptional range of motion, but most average adults are limited one way or another.

So as you start increasing your activities (like taking up a walking program or a jogging program), your biomechanics start functioning for or against you. What you find is that you might start getting little nagging aches and pains and injuries. An orthotic can help limit those discomforts, and balance you and help you reach your own unique, optimal position. Even though you might never be an elite athlete, you can be the B.E.S.T version of yourself by helping resolve this imbalance.

Orthotics and Exercise

Now that you're on my 30-day program, no doubt you are considering making a commitment to also start a regular exercise program. Set a goal for yourself and start thinking like an athlete in training. Maybe you want to run in a 10K or just make it around your neighborhood block without panting. You can achieve that goal without functionally breaking down. The biggest reason people give up on a new exercise regime is that they injure themselves to some degree, and it stops them—especially if they're not educated or they don't have someone helping them through this process. Arm yourself from the beginning and prevent any possible injury by educating yourself and becoming properly prepared. An orthotic is an excellent first step to insure that you are taking the proper precautions.

3

Mental Preparation

This program is a 30-day plan, but hopefully most everything you'll learn, you'll take with you for the rest of your life. There's a lot of mental preparation for going on the program, but even more importantly there's a mindset you'll develop for *staying* on it. My intent is to give you a plan you can live with. I've literally turned my passion for health into a career. Seeing results in my family, friends, and readers has kept me motivated to keep the information flowing.

Right now you're in the mindset that you want to make a change in your life. By reading this book, you are motivating yourself to get started. At the end of the 30 days, you're going to feel better than you do right this very minute. How's that for inspiration? One thing to really remember is that this program is not designed for a short-term quick fix. There is no magic pill you can swallow that will bring you to a state of total health. You have to do that yourself. You're not at some fancy spa where being healthy is made easy for you. You're in your own home, in your own environment. You can't pretend otherwise. Play around with the program a little bit. Experiment and see what works best for you. If you're someone who eats out all the time, know your prerequisites for that day's plan. You can live within the perimeters of this program because it's real food for real people living a real life. In fact, this program is full of helpful hints that I have discovered along the way to make my life easier.

You have to take responsibility for your health along the way. It's not up to anyone else around you. I'm going to help you make the right connection with the foods that you need, but it's up to you to use this program. There are no acceptable excuses for allowing anyone else (including ourselves) to sabotage our journey to total health. It's not just a weight issue. It's about self-esteem and self-exploration.

I have a friend who went on a liquid protein diet several years ago. She lost a significant amount of weight, but in such an unhealthy way. She looked thinner, but not healthy because her skin was pallid, her eyes lost their sparkle, and her whole presence had no vibrancy or glow. She had lost the weight so quickly and in such an unnatural way that it looked like her skin was hanging from her bones. Under all of that excess weight, there had been an angry woman who not only continued to live in her body, but also got angrier and angrier after her weight loss. For years she was able to hide the anger beneath the weight because she felt that being heavy didn't give her permission to express her feelings. Once she lost the extra pounds, she could no longer disguise those feelings, and in her own words, she turned into "a raving bitch." Not able to handle this flood of emotions that was flowing through her body, she decided it was easier to be fat and not have to deal with her anger than it was to be thin and deal with it.

There are lots of elements in our lives that threaten to sabotage us—the lack of availability of good food, lack of knowledge, other people in our sphere of influence, and the list goes on and on. As of this moment, that list should cease to exist. It's time to take responsibility for our own lives and to protect our health and ourselves.

Unlike those ads in the back of magazines, I'm not going to promise you that you will lose "30 pounds in 30 days." I will, however, promise that you are going to feel a lot better. You shouldn't think of this program as deprivation. It's more like a cleansing. It's like finally cleaning out your closet and finding some old clothes you haven't seen in years. (Or maybe finding clothes you didn't know you had.) This plan won't be the *end* for everyone trying to lose weight and get healthy, because it's really a beginning. It's about adjusting your perspective and your point of view on health. It is a very personalized plan because you will be taking control over what you choose to do. The more you practice this program, the more you'll *want* to practice this program. It's not a diet—it's a life plan.

This Is Not a Diet

If you read *Total Health Makeover* you know that I never think of myself as being on a diet. This program has become a way of life for me (and thousands of you, too). I am able to live this plan anytime, anywhere, under any extreme. Whether I was pregnant or on vacation, I never had to abandon the ten steps. The reason is that this program is exactly the way we were intended to eat. You'll find that the longer you're on my plan, the more you're going to want to stay on it because you feel so good.

You'll be reaping the benefits from the inside out and everyone will see how great you look and feel. What you'll learn from the next 30 days I hope you will take with you for the rest of your life. Sure, there'll be times that you fall off, but you will never be as far from your center as you used to be because you won't like that uncomfortable feeling of being out of balance. You're going to know the difference—maybe for the first time in your life.

When I first started practicing the principles laid out in this book, I would think of it as a diet. As soon as I would go on vacation, I would go off of it and blow it. Big time! When I'd visit my family I'd eat my way through Chicago, scarfing down an entire apple pancake from Walker Brothers Original Pancake House for breakfast, gobbling up a Maxwell Street Polish sausage for lunch, and inhaling an Uno's pizza for dinner. And you know what? I'd suffer the consequences. Bigger time! Pretty soon, I just didn't want to eat that way anymore because I didn't want to feel so lousy afterwards. And that's what I hope for you.

The Pleasure Principle

The pleasure principle is what makes the world go around. It's like eating and pro-creating—that's what we're here for, right? There's so much pleasure in those two natural functions of life, and I think it's so cool we get to do them so often.

Pleasure is what we're all looking for. Whether it's emotional or physical, we derive a certain sense of fulfillment from receiving (and giving) pleasure.

If people don't feel as if they're going to get pleasure out of something, they're not going to continue doing it. There has to be some hard work in there, but then you get a reward—and that is called pleasure.

I knew when I started getting healthy that I just couldn't live a Spartan life. I love to eat. There had been so many crazy diets that I used to go on where I couldn't enjoy my food. I was not having the pleasure of enjoying my meals on those diets, and when I broke them, I'd do it in such a stupid way that I would feel like "Oh my God, I blew it! I'm such a loser." (And I don't mean in weight.)

I love the food in this book. I love it. It's good food *and* it tastes good. It feels good on your tongue. It's sensual. It's life giving. It's got energy to it. It's got everything that good sex should have. It's life affirming. It's energetic. It's got a lot of flavors. The better you feel, the more alive you're going to feel. That's pleasure.

There's no way you can be in touch with being this animal that I keep talking about unless you know what it is you're supposed to be feeling. As you begin to live on this program, you'll start to feel a sense of pride that you have taken control of your health and well-being, and you'll be more organized. It's that sense of entitlement that says, "Yes! I deserve to be a sensual, healthy, life-giving person. I deserve to be full of energy and full of vibrancy."

"Once you start to take care of yourself, it feeds off itself and everything starts to fall into place. You start to take pride in how you look, what you're doing, where you're going, who you're with, how you affect people, what kind of energy you have, etc. It all reflects back to the pride and love you have for yourself. The outward messages that I send to the world come from a positive feeling that I have within."

—*Melissa Gomez, follower of the Total Health Makeover for four years*

I can look at people on certain diets and they look dead. They're walking around dead. They're vacant. There's no vibrancy to them. That friend of mine who went on the liquid protein diet looked like that. There's a healthy way to get healthy and there are unhealthy ways to lose weight. The difference is evident. Take a good look around you the next time you're out in the mall or standing in line at the movie theater. Do the people you see look healthy to you? If you don't like what *you* see in the mirror, don't break the mirror—change the reflection.

We know that we've got to find pleasure in whatever it is we do. Pleasure is what keeps us going. But like everything in life (and in my program), it's got to be balanced. What you have to do is find how to balance your pleasure with responsibility. That's why it is possible to find great joy and great pleasure in being responsible to yourself, to your children and family, and to your health. That's also why some of the happiest people are the people who really find real pleasure in their work. But when your pleasure meter swings so far out (and there's no responsibility to balance it), the equal and opposite reaction to it is going to be a shorter life because it probably has manifested itself as a drug or alcohol problem or as an eating disorder.

The pleasure of health is also about finding the pleasure of self—the pleasure of feeling good. The pleasure of having more energy, feeling sexier, more social, more in touch with your body and your life. More on top of things. Having the time to do the things you want to do. Less time wasted worrying about weight and health.

It's the pleasure of feeling you're at your optimum. It's the pleasure of feeling like you're ready to take on your day. No matter what the challenges are, you're ready to face them because you have a positive attitude and an extraordinary energy that says "I can handle it." You're no longer feeling run down by your health or your obsessive thoughts of being judged by your appearance. You know you're at your B.E.S.T.

This is what I call the pleasure of the *best* you. The pleasure of feeling you have control over temptations in your environment (bad food, bad habits, bad health). You *know* you're better than this. Something has made you interested enough to say it's time to change. That's what happened to me. I'm so excited because I feel like I have found a better way of living, and I plan on living a *very long time*. I've got two wonderful, adorable little boys, and I fully intend to be around for their weddings and to play with my grandchildren. And I want to have the kind of energy then that I have now.

Yet, even with all this "motivational pleasure," we still need the sense of reward. So that's why I'm building into this program certain special little foods that you love. This is probably the only program that recommends going out and having fun. In fact, toward the end of our 30 days together, I even suggest having a celebration dinner party.

Pleasure Foods

All foods should be a pleasure to eat, but there are certain foods that can be classified as "pleasure food." Pleasure foods are all those foods that are not the main foods of your diet that sustain life, but rather the extra filler foods that give you emotional satisfaction because they taste good, they're social, they're part of our culture. You know these foods, like cookies, candy, guacamole and chips, snack foods. (Yes, they're very much a part of my life, too.) The real problem is that a lot of people live *only* on pleasure food, and it can be a diet of empty calories.

On this program, you won't have to give up those foods that offer that kind of satisfaction. In fact, in the latter weeks, I've built in days where you get to sprinkle healthier versions of them throughout your day. You're not going to get them, however, in Boot Camp.

The idea is to put the kibosh on that mindless eating in front of a television set where it's just gut fill, and all you have is that empty bag of potato chips or container of ice cream. No question about it, we've all been there. Fun little pleasure foods are still going to be there on this program, but you're going to earn them. Isn't it true that we always have more satisfaction and take great pride (and pleasure) in the things we earn? I sure think so.

When I was experimenting with this program, I knew that I had to resolve the challenge of mixing my pleasure foods and remain true to my newfound way of life.

Eating is a great social pleasure to me, and yet I still wanted to look and feel the way I wanted without having a sense of deprivation. I finally got those two into balance. There were times when I may have had a momentary ounce of pleasure from bad food that was gratifying to me, but the sensation of waking up the next morning bloated and uncomfortable and not having anything to wear was just more trouble than it was worth. I knew that if I had to live the rest of my life picking at my food and feeling so deprived about the way I was eating, I'd always be battling pleasure and pain. I figured out how to get great pleasure from the food I now eat as well as have the pleasure of looking and feeling the way I want to. I know that this is why this way of life works.

The Difference Between "Getting There" and Maintenance

I have a few questions for you. How many times have you gone on some diet? How many times have you lost the same weight over and over again? How many times after gaining the weight you lost did you look for a new diet? We always know how to get there. We always know how to go on something short-term. I'm not looking for you to lose those extra pounds and then go back to your old ways. That's "getting there." We've all done that. What we now need to do is focus on staying there, and the only way you stay there is by making something that works a part of your life. The only way you stay there is by doing something that gives you enough health and energy. It's not just losing weight. It's how you got there that counts. Scale weight is not enough. What I'm hoping you come to at the end of these 30 days is not only losing some weight but changing your way of life. Think of it as every pound gone is gone forever and every unhealthy tissue gone is being replaced with new, improved, healthy tissue. I had spent years of yo-yo dieting as a teenager. After my mother's untimely death, I realized that it wasn't about my body and weight anymore, it was really about my health. That realization is what saved me not just in terms of health but also in terms of my inner struggle with battling my weight. Once I started being healthy, the weight fell off in an easier and more natural way than I ever dreamed possible. And it felt good. If you don't feel good doing something, then it's not going to be able to work long-term for you.

I'm making the assumption in this book that you've read the first book, and that you've tried the ten steps and have gone through your healing crisis already. Hopefully, you're seeing progress, but now you want a specific plan.

Falling in Love with the Process

In order to really "get there," you *must* fall in love with the process. If you do, "staying there" becomes second nature. It's so cool when you can fall in love with the process of just thinking about a new version of yourself. You can really throw yourself into it saying, "This isn't just going to be a short-term quick fix. I'm going to take this road, and it's going to lead me someplace wonderful. There may be some twists and turns, and it's going to be kind of bumpy for a while, but maybe I'll learn from my past, so that it will help me become the B.E.S.T version of me!"

I am looking for you to be able to add new things to your life. I don't know you. I don't know what you look like. I don't know where you've come from. I don't know how far away you are from this way of thinking. I do know that I would like you to take this road with me, and discover new things, and add to your life whatever works for you along the way.

If your goal is to get healthy, don't place a time limit on the process. Everyone is different. If at the end of our 30 days together you haven't reached your goal, don't throw your hands up in the air in frustration and stop practicing these ideas. Embrace the process and accept that you are most definitely better off than when you started.

Flexing the Discipline Muscle

I know a woman who is in her early forties who has been going through a tough time in her life. She has just gone through a divorce, and is living again with her parents. We were recently at the same wedding, and she told me that she had put on some weight and wasn't feeling particularly good about herself. She said she wanted to go on my program because she couldn't believe how much healthier I looked than when we first met 13 years ago. She said that she *wanted* to get healthy but didn't want to suffer for one day. She said, "I don't want to give up my dairy, my ice cream, my chips, any of my favorite foods."

Like this woman, many of us only think of healthy eating as a polite way of saying we're going to be deprived. We think of diets as deprivation rather than not really needing certain things. What if you didn't need that sugar and dairy anymore, and actually began to see it as a detriment? What if you had those foods once in a while but learned how to help your body recover from them quickly?

What I'm trying to get you to realize is that you can put a different spin on all of those old habits that clearly aren't making you happy. From everything this woman was telling me and from looking at her, I knew that she wasn't really happy with feeling the way she did.

It's all about turning that angle of the lens and having a new perspective that will help you flex that discipline muscle to stay on this program. One thing's for certain. Feeling deprived is never fun, but even deprivation can be viewed from a different angle. Try thinking of depriving yourself of old habits that have been controlling you as a *positive* thing. The only thing you're going to deprive yourself of on my 30-day program are those debilitating old habits that have been reigning over your life. That's how *I* think of deprivation on this program. Look at this as a liberation and a process of letting go of the old you and a rebirth of the new, better version of you.

When I first started on this journey, I might have thought, "Oh, I'm depriving myself of dairy and sugar and red meat and all these tasty foods that give me such pleasure." I had to retrain and rethink how I approached and tasted food. It's not like I went through some kind of hypnosis where those flavors did not appeal to me anymore. They just stopped appealing to me. The smell of cheese cooking is nauseating to someone who's given it up. It's like being a smoker. Many people derive a lot of pleasure from smoking. Once you're off cigarettes, you don't want a cigarette, or even if you do, you know that it's not good for you, and that's enough to keep you from smoking. You don't have that stink on your clothes anymore, and you don't have it on your breath. If you could make the same connection with bad food, you'll start to see what it is I'm saying. That's flexing the discipline muscle. It's focusing. It's challenging yourself to start thinking of things in a new way. It's saying to yourself, "I'm going to go through these five days of boot camp, and it's a little more disciplined than I'm used to being. I might have to cook a little bit more or cook a little less than I'm used to, but I'm going to just throw myself into it because this is boot camp, and it's basic training for the rest of my life."

Viewing Your Health in a New Way

When it comes to our health, why should we wait until it's too late to make changes that will affect how we spend our very limited time on this planet? Why should we wait until it's too late and we've got some kind of health problem? Wouldn't it be nice if we could gain control of these problems now? Think of this 30-day plan as *preventive* versus *prescriptive*.

You will learn all sorts of new things you never realized or even acknowledged in the past. I liken it to learning anything that's new. If you're learning to play the piano, you first have to learn to play the scales. Then one day all of a sudden you can play the piano. It's the same if you're warming up as a singer or doing your barre work as a ballerina. It's revisiting some of those basics. Since birth we've all been doing one thing: eating. Unfortunately, most of us have not been eating the right way. So now it's time to go back to some of the basics. Remember, Boot Camp is basic training for eating, because that's what it is. How can you be a good soldier and really fight the war unless you've been to Boot Camp and basic training? Similarly, how can your body defend itself unless it's been to Boot Camp and basic training?

I'm talking about our ability to defend ourselves through old age. I can't tell you how many people's bodies break down early because they never made the connection that it is due to their lifestyle habits. Don't we want to be vibrant and healthy right now? Why do we have to wait until we're old and infirm and trying to get ourselves back on the road? We're going to have a much harder job recovering after we've let ourselves go.

Why should we wait until it's too late? If you knew that something could improve the rest of your life, why wouldn't you want the rest of your life to start right now?

Changing Your Palate

As you start to become more aware of your body and the changes occurring every day, it's equally important to start to view your food in a new way too.

One of the things I talked about in *Total Health Makeover* is that I discovered early on in my newfound adventure of recreating myself and my health was that I never really took the time to taste my food. I would overly salt my meat or overly sugar my cereals, because those two flavors were the only two things my palate could taste. As I worked toward centering my diet and simplifying my food choices, I went on this kick of not only trying to taste the food I was eating, but also trying to dissect each and every aspect of it. If I ate an apple, I wanted to savor the taste of the meat, the skin, the core, and the juice individually. (In fact, I even ate the seeds, which are full of vitamins!) Together, these were the elements that made an apple taste like an apple. I wanted to know the difference in the flavors of each element. This experiment proved helpful in teaching me the principle of changing my palate or reprogramming my taste buds.

Do you really taste your food? When was the last time you actually tasted the simple grain flavors in a piece of bread? (Or do you need butter and jelly to give the bread any flavor?) Our tongues (or palate) have become so assaulted with the strong tastes of salt and sugar that they can't taste anything else. They have become anesthetized in a way to the more wonderful subtle flavors of the simpler foods that are not salted or sugared. Taste in food is very important. We all love food that tastes good, but our taste buds have become so destroyed that we can only taste extreme flavors. Certain extreme foods such as fats, meats, sweets, and processed foods will satisfy the immediate desire for certain tastes, but after a while, your taste buds become immune to tasting other flavors. In order to taste anything, the flavors have to become stronger and stronger.

How you taste food is important in creating balance in your diet. The first step to changing your palate is recognizing whether or not your palate has been numbed and your tongue swollen from years of extreme flavors and extreme foods. To change your palate, you have to eliminate the culprits causing the problems. On this program you'll be getting rid of your salt shaker at the table. Things will start to taste different to you because you will start to taste flavors other than "salt." If you have a sweet tooth, you won't be eating the sugary flavors that have been destroying your palate for years. When you do eat desserts you'll be eating ones that have been sweetened with natural sugars and are therefore less sickeningly sweet than refined sugar desserts. As you eliminate extreme foods and extreme flavors from your diet, you will eventually be able to rediscover foods that you haven't "tasted" in years.

What Kind of Eater Are You? The Seven Types of Eaters

I read in a Misho Kushi book (he's a teacher of macrobiotics) that he could define all eaters in one of seven categories. He explains The Seven Levels of Eating as mechanical eating, sensory eating, sentimental or emotional eating, intellectual eating, social eating, ideological eating, and free eating. This type of classification really struck a chord with me because I could relate to any one of those types at one time or another. It inspired me to come up with my own seven names based on these types of eating. They are the Robot, the Hedonist, the Crybaby, the Zealot, the Martyr, the Bargainer, and the Champion.

First, you've got the *Robot*. That's the automaton, the person who does mindless, automatic eating. They're not really enjoying it. It's just hand to mouth, the food goes in, they're not paying attention. They walk in, they've still got their coat on, they go to the refrigerator. There's no thought behind it. They're not listening to their body signals at all. We all know people who eat like this. (Or we've been known to eat like this.)

Next, there's the *Hedonist*. It's all about smells and tastes and textures. They could be stuffed, but as soon as they see or smell food, it's "Oh, I have to eat that. Oh my gosh. Oh, I'm stuffed but I can't stop myself. I want more and more because it's so good!" They're completely cued by outside signals. Every commercial sends them foraging in the refrigerator. They could be out to dinner and a movie, and upon entering the theater they buy the large bucket of popcorn no matter how full they are just because that's what they always do.

The *Crybaby* is the emotional eater who uses eating to stuff their feelings. They're the person who feels emotional about something, and they immediately don't want to have that feeling so they put it into the experience of eating. It's comfort eating. They're like Linus from *Peanuts*, but food is their blankie.

Then there's the *Zealot*, the person who does everything to the letter of the law. (This is not those of you reading this book. This is actually what I'm trying to get people away from.) A Zealot does not listen to what their own body is telling them. They follow a recipe so carefully that if it says 6 ounces it's not a fraction over or under that. Everything is measured and weighed and timed. They don't listen to their own internal signals, they're just doing everything obsessively according to the rules.

Next, there's the *Martyr*. This is the person who doesn't believe they're entitled to or deserve the best food. They're the ones who say, "Oh, you take the good piece." They don't eat well for themselves because God forbid they should treat themselves to anything. They're content with eating the bad piece of fish, the burnt piece of toast, or the smaller portion. They rarely sit down to enjoy their own plate of food and are happy scraping the leftovers from others. They don't put their needs first, because everybody else's needs come first.

Then there's the *Bargainer*. This is the person who bargains with their eating. You know, the person who says, "If I starve for three days, I can go crazy on the weekend." Or, "I'm going to diet to get in shape for something, and as soon as it's over, I'm going to really pig out." It's the feast or famine syndrome. They swing from one extreme to the other.

Finally there's the *Champion* eater. They eat according to the laws of nature, because they know it's the way that human beings should eat. They know how to listen to their own body signals. They're getting the right nutrition from their food.

They understand the proper quantities, and that sometimes it's going to be more, sometimes it's going to be less. It will always be based on what they're feeling at the time, not based on sensory clues or emotional clues, but what their body actually *needs*. Simply put, that's what we're trying to create in this book.

Dead Food Versus Live Food

Once you start to taste foods again in their purest form, you'll start to have a better understanding of the difference between "live" food and "dead" food. I always think of live food as something that gives you life. It has all of the right vitamins and nutrients in it naturally. Live foods are whole grains, fish, vegetables, fruits, and so on—anything that's going to be life giving.

Think of a live food in its raw state. As you take it further and further from its natural state, it becomes more and more dead. Dead foods are foods that have been overprocessed to the point of losing their vibrancy. You want to be sure to have as much vibrant live food as you possibly can.

For example, take something as common as a loaf of white bread. It's overprocessed, overmilled, overdenatured, overpasteurized, so far away from its live state that it's not going to add the same vibrancy to your health as something that's in its purer form. Sprouted whole-grain bread is going to be healthier than whole wheat, and whole wheat more alive than white bread. The further away you get from eating natural grains, the worse it is for your health. I eat grains every day. I definitely believe that you have to keep carbohydrates as part of your food pyramid. My carbohydrates tend to come in the form of grains rather than (overprocessed, overdenatured, overmilled) white flour carbohydrates. That's why I think oatmeal is so good for you. It comes in a pure state even though it's been cut, and it's an excellent source of grains and fiber.

If you eat a dead food diet of fast food, processed food, and junk food, it's all so chemicalized. Every single thing you eat is coated with fat or chemicals. Take your typical fast food burger. Each layer has some processing done to it (even the pickle).

The white bun has been milled down. The French fries are coated in oil. The hamburger is long dead. Now I'm not saying that everybody should eat only raw foods all the time and all their vegetables prepared without anything. That's boring. I'm just asking you to become more aware of the kinds of foods you're consuming.

Within the live foods, you want a certain amount of wet food, which is a subcategory. Wet foods help you digest concentrated foods such as a starch or a protein. The concentrated food is always going to take the most energy to digest, so eating a wet food will definitely help in the digestion process. For example, if you're having fish and a salad and vegetables for a meal, you want to make sure that at least one of your vegetables is steamed without adding soy margarine or oil. You want at least one clean, wet, live food per meal.

You've got to make your body work a little. If something is overprocessed, it will have fewer of the life-giving nutrients that your body needs.

Viewing Food in a New Way

Once you recreate your ability to taste food in its purest form and you comprehend the benefits of eating a live food diet (as often as possible), you will automatically start viewing what you eat in an equally new way. A fun way to remember what to eat is to apply my table seating theory to your food. A few years ago, I realized that when giving a party, every hostess is challenged to seat her guests so that she creates a perfect blend and balance for the evening. She has to think of all the different people coming to her party and must be absolutely certain that she creates a good mix at each table. People generally fit into one of four categories, and it doesn't have to be consistent. The same person can fit into a different category at a different dinner party.

The first type is your "anchor" or your "sun." It's the center person, the person that the rest of your table gets built around. It's usually the guest of honor or the person that everybody is driving to the party hoping they're going to talk to or sit next to. More often than not, the anchor is a sparkling raconteur whom everyone loves to listen to.

The second type is called the "swizzle stick." The swizzle stick is the person who mixes with everyone. A talk show host type, they know a little bit about each person and know how to go up to two people who don't know each other and say, "Oh, you two have something in common. . . ." They have a tendency to float the party, keeping sparkling conversation among all the different players.

The third type is your "chameleon." That's the person who blossoms and thrives or withers and dies depending on the person you seat them next to. You have to be very careful not to sit a chameleon next to the fourth type, which is your "wild card." This is the person you *don't* know who's coming to the party (someone has called and asked if it is okay to bring them), *or* it's the person you *do* know (often known as the "black hole")! They can sometimes be a real stick in the mud. You can't sit them next to an anchor or a chameleon so make sure you sit them next to a swizzle stick, because the swizzle stick won't let the circle of the party fall apart at that person. If you stick a chameleon next to a black hole, your table could die right there.

How Food Relates

So, I thought it would be fun to relate this analogy to the food that we eat. It's an unusual way to approach eating, but try it, it works! Your protein or starch entree is your anchor. It's the main attraction on your plate. Everything you eat has to work with that dish. Your green and non-starchy vegetables are the swizzle sticks because they mix with anything. Starchy vegetables are like a chameleon because they can either work for or against you. Anything you're avoiding from the ten steps, like dairy, sugar, meat, extra fat, is your black hole. Next time you're out to dinner with friends, tell them about this theory. At least you'll have fun trying to figure out who fits into each category and especially who the black holes are among the group!

4

A Recap and Update of the 10 Steps from Total Health Makeover

*I*n case any of you didn't read my first book (and for those of you who did), I want to briefly recap the ten steps I took to gain control of my health and become my B.E.S.T. Throughout my 30-day program, you will in fact practice most of the principles of all ten steps. With each stride, you will realize that your body is adjusting to its new routine. You'll find that you'll have more energy, and you're losing weight while eating more food than you ever thought possible. This is a program to retrain the way you think about food and how your body reacts to these changes. The important thing is to make a commitment to yourself to stay with the program I've designed for this book, and I promise you will see results. Even if you think you feel good right this minute, I assure you that 30 days from now you are going to feel even better! As I've already said, this is a program where the bad gets good and the good gets great!

The first step in taking better care of *you* is identifying what is right in your life. Take an honest look at the areas of your life that you feel good about and then at the areas that could stand some (or even lots) of improvement. Surely you know by now that there is no short-term solution to creating a long-term healthy life. Within these pages is a plan to help you get on that road to living a life that you are in control of instead of a life that controls you.

In *Total Health Makeover*, I explain that as you begin to restore your body to the animal it was meant to be, you can expect to encounter some bumps in the road. As you detoxify your system, it simultaneously begins to heal. Your body has to readjust itself to its new healthier existence. I refer to this process as the "Detoxification and Healing Crisis." It's the natural process your body will go through to undo the damage caused from years of abuse. A good example of this is the headache you may feel if you've ever tried to give up caffeine. The healing usually takes 3 to 4 days to cleanse your system, so it's not total torture. It's simply a physical reaction to the change in its environment. With each step you take, you may go through one or more physical reactions. The more out of balance your body is the more you may notice the process. This is a normal part of becoming healthy. Nothing can bring on this healing crisis without your body being willing to allow it to happen, so don't fear the change.

I would like you to feel really good about facing these challenges. With every step you take, you get one step closer to achieving that ultimate goal of finding a way of life that doesn't deprive you. A way that fills you with the satisfaction of knowing you are treating yourself the way you deserve to be treated—stronger, healthier, and with better clarity both physically and mentally. You will have boundless energy and an improved sense of total well-being. You won't be able to help but carry yourself a little differently, and I guarantee that everyone around you will say, "I want what you're having!"

Step One: The Dangers of Chemicals, Additives, and Preservatives

When is food not "real" food at all? For most people, the bulk of the food they eat is filled with chemicals, preservatives, and additives, which have no nutritional value and, to put it simply, are not foods at all. Of course, all of these additives are designed to do things to the food you eat like make it look better, help it last longer, and preserve it from spoiling. So many of the foods we eat were picked, canned, or shipped, a long time ago. Food manufacturers must put in these additives and preservatives in order to keep it looking fresh. Without these additives, many of the foods consumed on a daily basis would become inedible before they ever reached the supermarket shelves let alone our tables.

The average consumer eats about 140 to 150 pounds of food additives a year. This should clue you into the fact that we are putting substances into our bodies that aren't meant to be there. Most of the nearly 3,000 additives used in our food are not considered harmful by the FDA; however, that doesn't mean that they aren't doing damage to our bodies!

Consumers need to know the facts about chemicals, food additives, and preservatives. An educated eater is a healthy eater. The FDA defines additives as "any substance the intended use of which results or may reasonably be expected to result in affecting the characteristics of food." Chemical additives should be a frightening unknown to you. For example, pistachio nuts are not supposed to be red. (They're red because before industrialized farming, the nut pickers would sweat and stain the nuts. The distributor had to disguise the sweat stains with red dye.)

Do you really know what it is you're eating? We consume these chemicals in such great amounts, there's bound to be some side effects, whether or not you are aware of them. You have to learn to read labels so that you have a better understanding of what it is you are putting into your body. Additives can make you lethargic, sleepy, and wired, can cause headaches, and in worst case scenarios, cancer and other terminal diseases. Children especially, because of their low body weight, can have a reaction to these chemicals. Is it worth it? Of course, it's not realistic to think you can live a totally preservative or additive free life. Chemical preservatives in food, on a global level, have been a part of our life since World War II, when soldiers needed canned food to survive. They knew it wasn't healthy, but it was only meant to sustain life over a short period of time. After the war, the "convenience" of canned food took the country by storm, and became a popular modern way of eating in the fifties.

You can be more aware of cutting out those chemicals that have been proven to cause major side effects as a result of ingesting them. Just because the food is sold in the local supermarket doesn't mean it's safe. Preservatives are still added for the convenience of the retailer, but not for the well-being of us, the consumer. I personally don't want to eat anything that has a shelf life of one year. I say the fresher the pick, the better.

Step Two: Caffeine

What drug do four out of five Americans take on any given day? How about caffeine! It's found in coffee, tea, chocolate, cocoa, soft drinks, aspirin, and some analgesics commonly used for pain relief. Caffeine is in fact a drug, and can be highly addictive. It doesn't take much to develop a dependency on this drug. It is so readily available as an ingredient in many foods and drinks consumed every day. Caffeine is the most over-used stimulant in the world, and it can have a severe adverse effect on the nervous system. It is a drug that artificially elevates your mood and supposedly fights fatigue. To some, those may seem to appear as positive side effects, but recent studies show that caffeine can actually pose significant health risks, especially on unsuspecting susceptible people. It can cause hypertension, abnormal heart rhythms, problems with birth and/or pregnancy, osteoporosis, ulcers, heartburn, and panic and anxiety attacks. An overdose of caffeine can overstimulate your nerves, making you feel anxious, jittery, irritable, and even cause you to tremble. Too much caffeine can cause diarrhea and hot flashes.

Do you remember the first time you drank a cup of coffee? How did you feel? That reaction is still happening to you every time you drink a cup of coffee. We've become so desensitized to caffeine and its effects, we don't even notice. Can you imagine the toll it takes on your body over years of abuse? We have to ease up on the consumption to help eliminate long-term damage.

So what exactly is caffeine? Well, it's similar in structure to adenosine, which is a chemical found in the brain that actually slows down its activity. Since the two chemicals compete with each other, the more caffeine you consume, the less adenosine becomes available. But that's only temporary, so that explains the "high" you get from caffeine and why it only lasts so long. Within 30 to 60 minutes of drinking a cup of coffee, for example, caffeine will reach its peak penetration in the bloodstream. It typically takes 4 to 6 hours for those effects to wear off. Interestingly, coffee only accounts for three-quarters of the daily caffeine intake Americans consume. Tea, soft drinks, and chocolate make up most of the remaining 25 percent. In fact, did you know that 8 ounces of Dannon coffee yogurt packs the same caffeine punch as a 12-ounce can of Coke? Obviously, you can take in extreme amounts of caffeine even if you don't drink coffee, so it's important to read those labels!

There's the good, the bad, and the ugly when it comes to caffeine. While it is true that you can get a quick jolt of energy from drinking a cup of coffee, it doesn't last very long and often you'll find yourself jittery and nervous from the caffeine. If you drink too much caffeine, you can find yourself unable to fall asleep. It can overstimulate the nerves, making you feel restless, anxious, nervous, and irritable. The amount of caffeine needed to trigger a reaction depends on your own sensitivity to the drug and how often you drink it. Some people have very few side effects from caffeine, while others, especially if they're not used to it, can have a major reaction from the slightest amount. Caffeine can also cause facial flushing, diarrhea, and frequent urination. People with high blood pressure should avoid caffeine altogether, because it can raise blood pressure. It doesn't take much to develop a dependency on caffeine either. One study shows that 1 to 3 cups of coffee a day will do it. The average cup of coffee (6 ounces) typically supplies around 100 mg of caffeine. Within 30 to 60 minutes of drinking a cup of coffee, caffeine reaches its peak concentrations in the bloodstream. It usually takes 4 to 6 hours for its effects to wear off.

The average adult consumes around 200 mg of caffeine a day and the top percentage of those people take in more than 400 mg a day! Even at 200 mg a person is on his or her way to distress. Drinking more than 600 mg a day can lead to stomach ulcers, hand tremors, an irregular heartbeat, and insomnia. Caffeine promotes stomach acid secretion, so it can be a potentially dangerous substance for those with peptic ulcers.

How do you know if you're dependent on caffeine? Try eliminating all caffeine from your diet for one day. See how you feel. If you get a throbbing headache, you're probably drinking too much caffeine. The intensity of withdrawal is usually equal to the amount of addiction. Quitting caffeine can have some pretty significant side effects. The most common complaint is a frequent headache. One study showed that 10 percent of the volunteers who quit caffeine went through severe withdrawal symptoms. They became depressed, fatigued, and some even complained of flu-like symptoms including nausea and vomiting. In general, the symptoms appear within 12 to 24 hours after kicking the habit, and virtually all caffeine in your body is eliminated during that time. The withdrawal symptoms seem to be the worst on the first or second day and can last up to a week, although the usual time is four days. You can quit cold turkey or gradually wean yourself off of caffeine. You have to decide what you can handle. If you only drink coffee in the morning, the craving you have first thing in the morning for that cup may actually be a withdrawal symptom. Sometimes people only drink coffee during the week, so on the weekends, they might suffer some withdrawal-like symptoms. But coffee, although the most commonly thought of source of caffeine by people, isn't the only culprit. About 2 to 4 cans of caffeinated soda or 2 to 4 cups of tea can provide as much caffeine as a cup or two of coffee. A cup of black tea (it's the most common tea in America) supplies around 50 mg of caffeine. Green tea and oolong tea have much less caffeine, and herbal teas don't have any. Seventy-five percent of the caffeine contained in tea seeps through the tea in the first 30 seconds of brewing. Eight of the ten best-selling brands of soda all contain caffeine. Most of these contain 35 to 45 mg of caffeine, but there are some that are much higher. The kola-nut extract used to flavor colas naturally contains caffeine. Manufacturers say that they add caffeine to balance out the sweetness, but the real reason is to keep you drinking their products. Chocolate contains caffeine because the cocoa-bean powder used to make the candy contains natural caffeine. An average chocolate bar contains around 30 mg. One of the most surprising places that hide caffeine is in everyday medications. Manufacturers can add as much as 100 mg of caffeine to certain cold medicines, muscle relaxers, pain-relievers, and anti-migraine drugs. So if you're popping back a couple of aspirin every four hours, you could be taking in a hefty dose of caffeine in the process.

Caffeine can be hard on your bones. The more caffeine a woman drinks, the more calcium is excreted in her urine. She is losing an extra 5 mg of calcium for every 6 ounces of coffee or two cans of soda. The FDA banned the use of caffeine in over-the-counter weight loss drugs in 1991. It had no long-term effect on weight. It is still used in aspirin and other painkillers, however. Caffeine increases their potency by 40 percent.

Caffeine is found in so many different products that merely switching to decaffeinated coffee won't solve the issue for you, but it will help reduce your intake if you can't bear the thought of leading a coffee-free life. Read nutritional labels on everything and go for the brands that are caffeine free whenever possible. If you do decide to eliminate caffeine from your life, wean off it slowly if you start to get painful headaches. You will win the battle of the bean if you stick with it.

Step Three: Sugar/Sugar Substitutes

I recently appeared on the *Donny & Marie* show with my two young sons. Nicky, my older child, was offered a piece of candy during the program, and he graciously declined, telling Donny, "No thank you, I don't eat sugar." A few days later, I received the following e-mail on my website.

Dear Marilu,

I was just watching the **Donny and Marie** show and you were on with your son Nicky. Donny broke a piñata open and afterward offered a pack of candy to your son. He refused, saying that he doesn't eat sugar.

Boy . . . I was drinking a Coke at the time from Taco Bell. That inspired me to dump out the drink and refill my cup with water, ice, and a touch of orange juice for flavor.

Thank you for giving me the inspiration!

Sindy Verdugo Cox
Nicky's First Convert!

Getting caught up on a sugar treadmill is dangerous, especially for children. I have often referred to sugar as "kiddy cocaine," because in my opinion, that is exactly what it is. Watching your child's behavior change right before your very eyes from eating sugar can be a very dramatic experience. It is like giving the child a drug. It stimulates, causes mood swings, and can be addicting. Sounds like a drug to me! Giving your child sugar is such an unhealthy food choice. It only stimulates and trains him or her toward unruly and unhealthy behavior.

Americans consume somewhere in the neighborhood of *136 pounds of sugar per person, per year.* Sugar adds calories to your daily intake, and those are often "empty" (meaning no nutritional value) calories. Over half of the sugar consumed today is added directly from the sugar bowl while eating or preparing a meal. The food manufacturers add the other half, either as sugar or as high-fructose corn syrup. Your body breaks down sugar that you eat into the sugar found in the blood, called glucose.

In recent years, refined white sugar has been blamed for diseases such as hyperactivity, diabetes, hypoglycemia, bad moods, yeast infections, obesity, and tooth decay. Refined white sugar depletes your body of all of the B vitamins. It leaches calcium from your hair, blood, bones, and teeth. It interferes with the absorption of calcium, protein, and other minerals in your body, and retards the growth of valuable intestinal bacteria.

Sugar has a fermenting effect in your stomach. It stops the secretion of gastric juices and inhibits the stomach's ability to digest. Sugar is not digested in the mouth like other foods. When eaten alone, it passes directly into the small intestine, but when eaten with other foods, it sits in the stomach for a while. Sugar in the stomach is a sure way to guarantee rapid acid fermentation in the warm and moist conditions of the stomach. So, drinking a regular soda with your meal or sugar in your coffee while eating breakfast definitely ignites that fire.

Kicking the sugar habit isn't an easy thing to do. I know that when I decided to give up sugar, it was a difficult decision for me. My theory on this one is that once you start eating sugar, you want more and more of it, even if your stomach tells you it's full.

(That's the sugar treadmill.) It goes beyond satisfying a simple urge. People generally eat to fill their stomachs, not caring what they put into it. But you should care, because so much of how we feel and think and act is tied to what we eat, right?

If you want to get off that sugar treadmill, try cutting down on your total sugar intake. Eliminate all added sugars and decrease your intake of foods that are high in sugar. It's that simple. And on this program, you will eat only foods that are naturally sweetened.

I found that when I gave up sugar, I also ended up giving up red meat (step four). They are total opposites in terms of being yin (sugar) and yang (meat). The reason you crave one with the other is that they balance each other out because they're both so extreme on the food number line—the line on which all foods are placed from extreme yin (expansive) to extreme yang (contractive). Dropping both from your diet makes it easier to stick with not eating either food, because your craving for both goes way down. The more vegetable protein you eat in place of animal protein, the lower your desire for sugar will be. That craving for something sweet after you eat simply fades after a while because you're eating a much more balanced meal.

Once you decide to kick the sugar habit, you'll notice that your taste buds will start picking up flavors and sensations you may have never experienced before. Everything you eat will start to taste better and more alive in its flavor. Oddly enough, it's not the food that tastes better, it's your body that's better able to taste the food. (You'll find that this is a common side effect when choosing any one of my ten steps.)

Healthy Substitutes for Sugar

My intent in giving up sugar is not to take the sweet temptation out of your life, but rather to improve the quality of your health and food choices. If you're ready to give up sugar, then I suggest clearing out all of the food items in your home that might be a temptation. Get rid of the candy bars, the cookies, and that ice cream. Here's the good news. You can get healthy sugar-free substitutes for practically every item in your cupboards, refrigerator, and freezer (and I'm *not* talking about chemical-laden sugarless substitutes made with aspartame and saccharin!). If you drink coffee with sugar and/or milk, my suggestion is to get rid of all three things. I know some of you are very attached to that cup of Joe, so try using raw honey as a sweetener. Better yet, use "Rice Dream" rice milk, which is slightly sweet. You could always switch to flavored herbal tea, which is easy to drink without any added sweetener.

Replacing sugar with raw honey is a good idea, but be aware that honey is more concentrated than white sugar (see chart below). You only need to use half the amount of honey that you would sugar. Honey gets assimilated into the bloodstream very quickly, and it has certain minerals and enzymes that don't upset the body's mineral balance as much as sugar does. Honey was used as medicine for centuries. It has natural properties that can have a healing effect on the liver, neutralize toxins in the body, and even work as a pain reliever. If you eat mostly a grain and vegetable diet, a small amount of honey is usually enough to satisfy your taste needs. If you use honey, go for raw, completely unprocessed, unheated honey.

The least concentrated, least sweet, and the closest to being a whole food sugar substitute are products that contain maltose. They are one-third as sweet as white sugar and are not highly processed. Rice syrup and barley malt are primarily maltose and are very easy to find in the health food store. One of the main reasons I recommend these as an excellent substitute is that at least half of the composition of the grain-based sweeteners are nutrients found in whole grains. They also take longer to digest in the stomach. That helps even out blood-sugar peaks and valleys that highly refined sugar can cause. If you've never tried rice syrup or barley malt, you'll be trying them in this program. They're really good tasting, easy to use in recipes, and extremely easy to get used to.

Chemically Processed Sweeteners

Sweetener	*Source*
White sugar	Cane and sugar beets
Raw sugar	Cane and sugar beets
Brown sugar	White sugar with molasses added

Corn syrup	Processed from corn starch
Blackstrap molasses	By-product of granulated sugar (contains minerals)

Fructose, xylitol, and sorbitol can be made from natural sources, but it is too expensive, so they are refined from commercial glucose and sucrose. Read label for source.

Naturally Processed Sweeteners

Sweetener	Composition Source
Unrefined sugar	Unrefined cane juice powder
Maple syrup	Boiled-down sugar maple tree sap
Sorghum molasses	Cooked-down cane juice
Barbados molasses	Cooked-down cane juice
Rice syrup and barley malt	Fermented grains—less destructive to the body's mineral balance
Honey	Nectar from flowers processed in the stomach of bees
Fruit juices	Fruit
Fruit syrups and date sugar	Fruit—far more concentrated and sweeter than fresh fruit
Amasake	Fermented rice maltose

Step Four: Meat

Hello Marilu!

I bought your book a few months ago when I was traveling for work. My husband and I have now eliminated red meat and dairy from our diet. Since August, I

have lost 13 pounds and my husband has lost 18. I have never eaten more healthy foods, and I really feel great!

Laura Pitaniello

Humans were meant to be primarily vegetarian. Our closest living relatives from the animal world, apes, are vegetarians. Even cows are, by nature, vegetarians. (We're just getting their healthy grass and grain diet once removed!) The structures of our skin, teeth, stomach, bowels, and the length of our digestive system are all typical of vegetarians. Somewhere along the way, we overcame our physical limitations and decided to kill other animals for food. If you took away all modern technology which slaughters, butchers, and delivers meat to our local grocery store, it would be filled with nothing but fruits and vegetables—the foods God intended for us to eat. Of course, you can survive quite easily on a diet that consists of no animal products, often referred to as a vegan diet. Most of the world's human population is largely vegetarian. Despite the information that is put out by the Meat and Livestock Commission, humans do not need meat. People always say, "I don't feel strong when I don't eat meat. Meat gives me strength." The largest and strongest dinosaur was a vegetarian. A chimpanzee is a vegetarian. Eating meat has nothing to do with strength. In fact, it zaps your strength because it overtaxes your digestive system and wears you out. Eating meat, especially red meat, is associated with promoting your risk of cancer. People who eat red meat five or more times a week are four times more likely to have colon cancer than people who eat no meat or eat it less than once a month. Women who eat beef, lamb, or pork as a daily main dish are two and a half times more likely to develop colon cancer than women who eat meat less than once a month. The substitution of other protein sources such as beans and lentils is known to reduce the risk of colon cancer. Prostate cancer is another risk.

Meats are higher in animal fat, which is harder for us to digest and therefore stays in our bodies longer. The human digestive system wasn't meant to break down the flesh from another animal.

People ask me all of the time whether or not I eat chicken. When I first started this program, I didn't intend to give up chicken. But about two and a half years after giving up red meat, chicken started to taste funny to me. Its texture seemed way too hard to digest and the smell and taste just didn't appeal to me anymore, so I gave it up. At that time there were also very few "free range" chicken products available. Today, I still don't eat chicken, and I don't really recommend it in the long run for women because it is too concentrated a protein for females. My husband and sons eat a little chicken as long as it is free range. It's important that the chicken is free range because the chicken is raised on natural grains and allowed to run free as opposed to being shot with steroids and growth hormones and cooped up in a tiny cage.

Step Five: The Miracle of Dairy Free

Marilu—

Seeing your before and after pictures, and reading what you had to say about dairy made so much sense to me. I stopped all dairy and lost weight. My face cleared up completely. Your book is like a bible to me that I can read and refer to whenever I need an extra boost. Especially when I run into people who think I'm crazy for not eating dairy products. Thank you, Marilu, for being my catalyst.

Cindy Nervino
California

I have been virtually dairy free since 1979, and believe me when I tell you unequivocally that eliminating dairy from your diet will change your life forever. It'll change the way you look, how you feel, and add years to your life. Almost every single person I talk to about this program invariably says to me, "There is no way I could ever give up milk or cheese." The overwhelming response from everyone is that they might be able to deal with all of the other aspects of this health makeover, but the dairy thing, well, that just seems downright impossible! I should know. When a nutritionist first suggested (based on my family history and what he could "read in my face") that I give up dairy, I was one of those people! After reading about the connection between dairy and heart disease and dairy and arthritis, I decided, "What the hell, I'll try it for three months."

I used to love cheese, especially Jarlsberg and Brie. In fact, I loved dairy so much that I used to buy "cheese ends" at my local gourmet food shop. So less than three months later (I couldn't even go the distance, that's how addicted to dairy I was), I decided I just had to have a night of unabashed Jarlsberg. I ate three big bites of it, and I thought, "Oh my God! This is like eating my shoe!" It just tasted disgusting to me. The smell was funny (like feet), and the consistency was weird. Once I finally got off dairy for good, my face changed so much. That baby fat layer brought on and carried because of dairy consumption went away. I had bone structure that I never had before. My lungs and kidneys were functioning better because they got unclogged from that dairy sludge that was blocking their function.

Everyone who goes off dairy talks to me about having more energy, better digestion, and feeling less stuffy in their nose. I can't think of anyone who didn't feel a difference. They might not stay completely dairy free, but they never go back to where they were as far as how much dairy they used to eat. They know in the back of their heads that they shouldn't be eating dairy.

I'm always saying that the only thing milk is supposed to do is to turn a 50-pound calf into a 300-pound cow in six months. If cows don't drink milk, why would we? If I offered you a cold glass of breast milk, would you drink it? Okay, maybe you might, but what if I offered you dog's milk or orangutan's milk? (Frankly, it makes more sense that we would drink orangutan milk, because we are closer to them as a species than we are to a cow.) Humans were never meant to consume anything other than human breast milk, and only while we're babies. We are the only animals on earth that drink the milk of another animal. Milk is a food of convenience, and in our quest for convenience, we have made ourselves one of the sickest animals on the face of the earth. In many countries, the thought of drinking milk from a cow is as absurd as drinking milk from an orangutan. Milk is nature's food for a baby calf, which has four stomachs, and will double its weight in 47 days. Not only does a baby calf have four stomachs, it also has 9 feet of intestines as opposed to humans, who have 27 feet of intestines. Our digestive enzymes are not capable of breaking down a food that is designed to nurse the young of another species. Our stomachs don't even recognize dairy as a "food," and everything we eat with it has a difficult time digesting in the process.

Maybe you're thinking to yourself, "What about all of the good things we hear about milk, like it helps provide calcium and keeps our bones strong?" Although millions of dollars are spent every year lauding the virtues of milk, the truth is that the calcium in cow's milk is much coarser than in human milk, and the human body does not adequately absorb it. Also, all of the processing of dairy products reduces the calcium supply in those products, so it becomes very difficult to use pasteurized, homogenized, or other processed dairy products as a good source of calcium. In fact, most of us could get enough calcium through other foods we eat, so we don't need to get it from milk. Salmon and soy products are excellent sources of calcium. Spinach, broccoli, and all other green leafy vegetables contain calcium. Nuts and sesame seeds are also great sources of calcium. Even concentrated fruits like dates, figs, and prunes offer enough calcium for your body's needs. Cows get their calcium from eating grass in the fields where they graze.

Making butter requires 21.2 pounds of milk for each "finished" pound of butter. One quart of milk weighs 2.15 pounds. The fat found in dairy products is animal fat, which is high in cholesterol. Whole milk and anything made from whole milk is very high in saturated fat, which can increase your cholesterol level. "Saturated" is a chemical term that means the fat molecule is completely covered with hydrogen atoms. Without those atoms, the fat is "unsaturated." Saturated fats stimulate your liver to make more cholesterol. Most animal products contain substantial amounts of saturated fat. Lose dairy, and you'll lose fat. (For more information about fat, see step seven on "fat.")

The Miracle of Soy

One of the reasons that soy products are used so much as dairy substitutes is because tofu has a consistency very similar to dairy. Hopefully, by the time you've started this program, you've already weaned yourself off dairy. Some of you may have a problem cleaning out the dairy residue lingering in your body. We're going to try and keep the meals as simple as possible in the beginning of this program. Legumes will not be introduced until well into the second week (especially soy, because of its similarity to dairy). It's best to get off dairy completely, cleanse your system, and then introduce soy-based foods.

If you're basically allergic to dairy, and you've been eating a lot of it, you shouldn't go right to soy substitutes, because soy and dairy are so closely connected that you may have to not eat either for a little while until you "clean out the dairy." I saw a nutritionist who explained to me that I was so allergic to dairy that my body was being tricked into believing that the soy was the same thing. Dairy was such a staple of my diet that I was still holding on to the leftovers. He suggested that I not eat any soy for one month and really let my system flush out the dairy. He explained to me that I should eat pineapple three times a week for breakfast because the bromelain in it would help "dissolve the dairy." This nutritionist said that at around the third or fourth week I would eat the pineapple, and it would taste too strong and acidic for me. That's when I would know that it was safe to reintroduce the soy products into my diet. Sure enough, around three and a half weeks in, I was having pineapple and I just couldn't eat it anymore. I would recommend that if you have been a heavy dairy eater, try eating pineapple for a few weeks so that your body isn't tricked into thinking you're still eating dairy.

We all know that milk comes from a cow, but where do "soy" products come from? There are three types of soy protein, all of which are derivatives of the soybean. These include Soy Protein Concentrate, Isolated Soy Protein, and Textured Soy Protein. The Isolated Soy Protein is the greatest source of pure soy, containing 92 percent protein. Soy protein is a complete source of protein containing all essential amino acids needed for the human body to build and maintain healthy muscle tissue.

In fact, eating soy products has been linked to helping osteoporosis and menopause. Three recent studies have found that peri-menopausal women experience improvements in negative menopausal symptoms such as hot flashes, higher cholesterol, and elevated blood pressure by using soy supplements. Interestingly, symptoms such as hot flashes are very uncommon in women from countries where the consumption of soy products is high, such as Japan and other Asian countries. In fact, there is no word in Japanese to translate "hot flash"!

In the first three to five years after menopause, women lose 3 to 5 percent of their bone mass *per year*. After ten years, bone loss tapers off. The isoflavins in soy have been found to have a positive effect on bone tissue in recent studies. John J.B. Anderson recently confirmed this theory in his review entitled "The Effects of Phytoestrogens on Bone" in the journal *Nutrition Research*. He agreed that findings show that at optimal doses, soy-based isoflavins showed an improvement in bone mass. It's a good idea to eat soy products daily instead of taking isoflavin supplements. Additionally, make sure you're getting enough vitamin D and calcium in your diet and exercising regularly to protect yourself against the threat of osteoporosis. (There's calcium in soy products as well.) Soy is now such a staple in my diet that there isn't a day that goes by without my eating it in some form. In fact, the one thing you will always find in my refrigerator is a large bowl of cooked soybeans (edamame). I buy bags of them frozen at the health food store and I pop them in boiling, lightly sea-salted water for five minutes. Everyone in my family loves them. In fact, my kids eat them like they're M&Ms.

Step Six: Food Combining

Dear Marilu:

After reading your book, I am giving up dairy and am now food combining. This is just my second week into your program, but I feel better already. I never walk away from a meal feeling as if I've over-eaten. I just feel satisfied. Your book has been greatly appreciated!

Susan Wilkins
Maryland

I have turned more people on to food combining who can't get over how simple yet effective it is. I have also received thousands of e-mails from people who have adopted this way of eating who now swear it works. The basic idea is to think of your meals as either a fruit, a starch, or a protein meal. At first, it seems like an unusual way to approach eating, because it was the exact opposite of the typical American diet, which is a "meat and potatoes, spaghetti and meatballs, turkey sandwich" way of life. Most "diets" recommend a protein exchange, a bread exchange, and a fruit exchange for dessert, which contradicts the basics of food combining. They do this to purposely keep you feeling full.

Not only do I believe that proper food combining is the healthiest way to eat, but you end up losing weight and having more energy in the process. This isn't a diet about counting calories or about portion control. It's a program that teaches you to respect the chemical properties of each food and how each food reacts when combined with other foods.

When I first started food combining, I would let my mind wander and made up meals in my head that stayed within the rules. It was hard to believe that it could actually work. I'd have an all-starch night at a favorite Italian restaurant that included potatoes, pasta, vodka, and bread. I tried an all-fish night in which I ate smoked salmon as an appetizer, grilled swordfish for dinner, and a salad with tuna sashimi for dessert. To my shock and total amazement, it worked! I knew that this was *a lifestyle change* and not just another fad diet.

After trying food combining for a while, I felt lighter and more balanced and I wanted to feel that way forever. I felt stronger, I stood up straighter, and I really felt better about myself. Believe me, it showed in *everything* I did. The amount of weight that I lost was incredible, and the weight loss came naturally with all of the other benefits. If you perfectly food combine, you won't believe the results. Your digestion will work so much better, and the volume of food you can eat will surprise you. You lose that gassy, bloated, stomach-distended feeling. Suddenly, your food starts working for you, not against you.

Everything you will read and hear about food combining makes it sound so logical that it will seem incomprehensible that you don't already live your life that way. The principles of a proper food combining diet are easy to follow once you have a grasp of the basics. The best thing is that you get to eat more food than when you are on a "typical diet," but you'll be eating less food than when you pig out. It allows you to eat more volume on a daily basis, but not in that feast or famine, crazy out-of-control way.

When protein and starches are eaten together, it takes so much energy to digest that meal. The body gets confused and cannot manufacture the necessary enzymes at the same time to properly digest the food. Undigested food just sits in the stomach for hours, rotting and unable to properly digest, which creates toxins in the bloodstream. Some digestion *does* take place, but particularly through bacterial action, which causes fermentation. This fermentation is the cause of such side effects as gas, bloating, and abdominal pain. Bacterial digestion creates another important side effect, poisonous by-products such as ptomaine and leucomaine. Bacterial fermentation of starch can also result in toxic by-products like acetic acid, lactic acid, and carbon dioxide. Proper food combining helps the body digest enzymatically, which produces essential amino acids that repair and maintain the body. Proper food combining ultimately enhances the nutritional value of the well-digested food. When we eat the *wrong* foods together the result is digestive trouble. We're so used to feeling lousy after a meal (stuffed, bloated, and gassy) that unless we feel that way, we don't feel we've eaten! Eating certain foods together interferes with digestion, which ultimately leads to poor health and unwanted excess pounds. Eating "starch-rich" foods in combination with "protein-rich" foods is the most common mistake people make in their diet. Avoiding this mistake is the underlying premise behind food combining because eating proteins and starches together unnecessarily taxes the digestive system. Proteins and starches require different digestive enzymes, which function at different pH levels in the body. Pepsin digests protein in the highly acidic environment of the stomach. Starches prefer alkaline environments such as the intestines. Combining these two types of food traps them and slows down the digestive process. The undigested food is what causes the digestive problems such as gas, bloating, constipation, and weight gain.

Food combining does not limit your choices in terms of what to eat, but only in what to eat *together* for the best results. I really believe that food combining is the healthiest approach to eating you can take. It's not a diet in the traditional sense because it allows you to eat a healthier amount of food than most other programs.

My food-combining program is designed to offer you the most effective method for digestive excellence. It is based on the same principles and eating patterns that our earliest ancestors lived by. Almost all of the meal plans for this 30-day program will follow this practice of eating the right foods together. This simple approach to eating is a return to the basics and the way our bodies were meant to eat and digest.

One really simple way to understand why food combining works is a lesson in Chemistry 101. Imagine your stomach as a beaker. When you eat a protein (fish, chicken, meat, eggs, dairy), your mouth sends a signal to the brain to put an acid base in the stomach in order to digest the protein. When you eat a starch (bread, potatoes, rice, pasta, grains), the mouth sends a different signal to the brain to send an alkaline base to digest it. The reason you don't want to be eating proteins and starches together is because ACIDS AND ALKALINES NEUTRALIZE EACH OTHER! Nothing gets properly digested. It's scientific. We derive no nutritional value from undigested food. In fact, food that is left undigested just rots in our stomachs. The rotting causes a toxic response by turning into poison and alcohol, leaving us with a toxic mess to clean up. Once we eat, food has two choices. It either digests or it doesn't. Proper food combining leaves you with only one choice and that is proper digestion. It also sets a stage for more energy and less weight. You will realize how wonderful food combining feels firsthand once you try it.

The following is your best guideline to food combining and the rest of "The Rules":

The Basic Rules of Food Combining

1. Do NOT eat proteins and starches together. Your body requires an acid base to digest proteins and an alkaline base to digest starches. Proteins and starches combine well with green, leafy vegetable and non-starchy vegetables, but they do not combine well with each other.

Marilu Henner's Food-Combining Chart
Chart 1

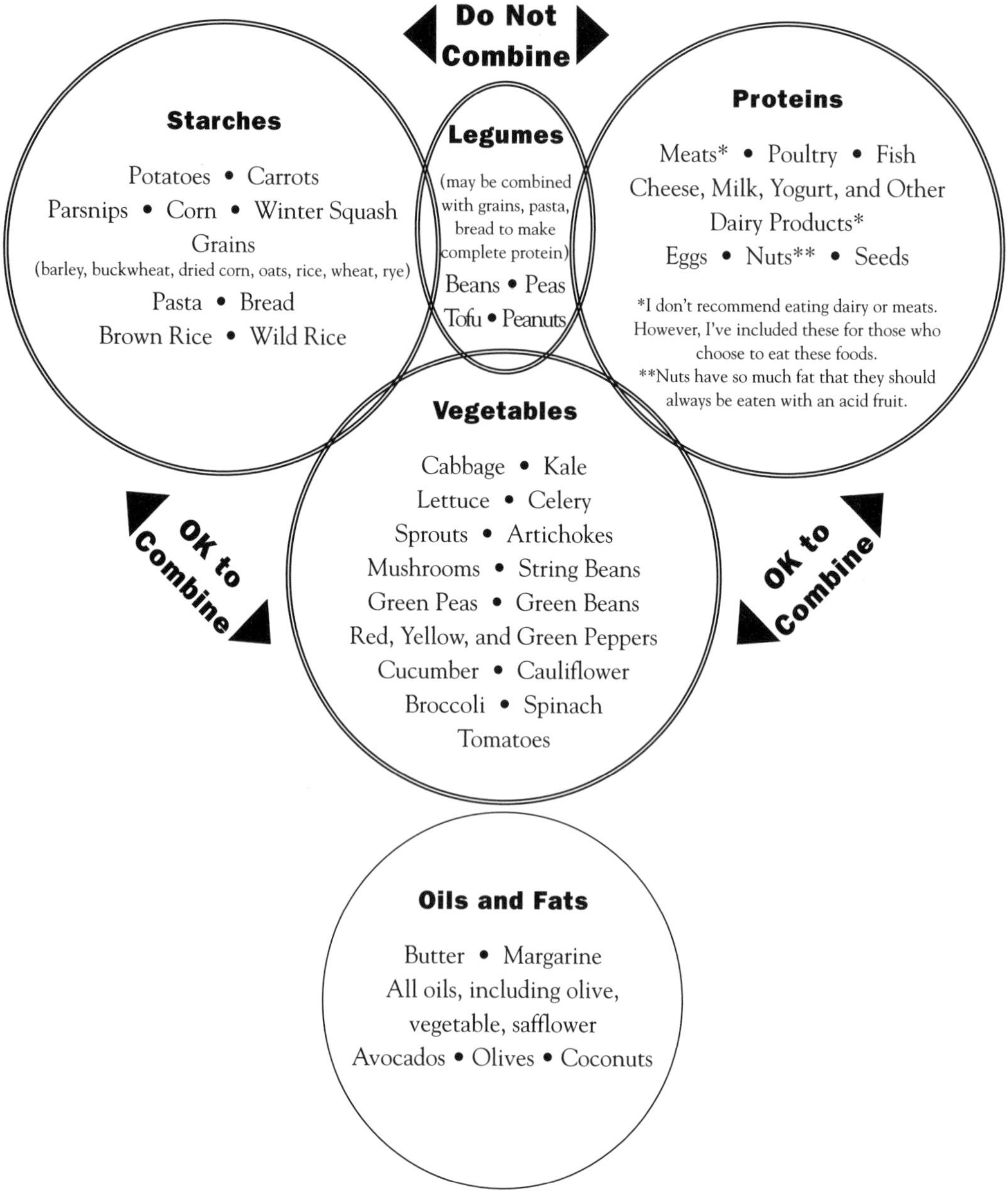

◄ Do Not Combine ►

Starches

Potatoes • Carrots
Parsnips • Corn • Winter Squash
Grains
(barley, buckwheat, dried corn, oats, rice, wheat, rye)
Pasta • Bread
Brown Rice • Wild Rice

Legumes

(may be combined with grains, pasta, bread to make complete protein)

Beans • Peas
Tofu • Peanuts

Proteins

Meats* • Poultry • Fish
Cheese, Milk, Yogurt, and Other
Dairy Products*
Eggs • Nuts** • Seeds

*I don't recommend eating dairy or meats.
However, I've included these for those who
choose to eat these foods.
**Nuts have so much fat that they should
always be eaten with an acid fruit.

Vegetables

Cabbage • Kale
Lettuce • Celery
Sprouts • Artichokes
Mushrooms • String Beans
Green Peas • Green Beans
Red, Yellow, and Green Peppers
Cucumber • Cauliflower
Broccoli • Spinach
Tomatoes

◄ OK to Combine ►

◄ OK to Combine ►

Oils and Fats

Butter • Margarine
All oils, including olive,
vegetable, safflower
Avocados • Olives • Coconuts

Do Not Combine Foods from Charts 1 and 2
Chart 2

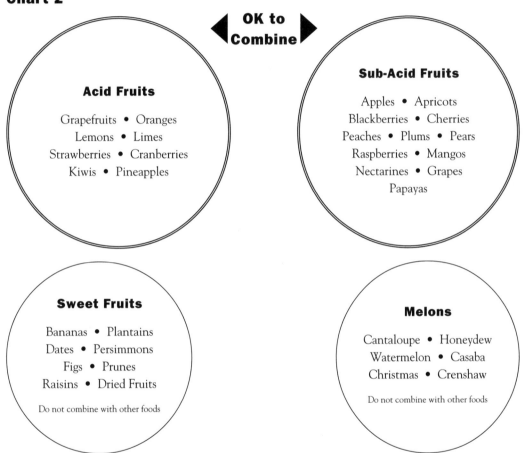

OK to Combine

Acid Fruits

Grapefruits • Oranges
Lemons • Limes
Strawberries • Cranberries
Kiwis • Pineapples

Sub-Acid Fruits

Apples • Apricots
Blackberries • Cherries
Peaches • Plums • Pears
Raspberries • Mangos
Nectarines • Grapes
Papayas

Sweet Fruits

Bananas • Plantains
Dates • Persimmons
Figs • Prunes
Raisins • Dried Fruits

Do not combine with other foods

Melons

Cantaloupe • Honeydew
Watermelon • Casaba
Christmas • Crenshaw

Do not combine with other foods

2. Do NOT mix fruit with proteins, starches, or any kind of vegetable. Fruits digest so quickly that by the time they reach your stomach they are already partially digested. If they are combined with other foods, they will rot and ferment. *Only* eat fruit with other fruits.

3. Melons digest faster than any other food. Therefore, you should NEVER eat melons with any other food, including other fruits. Always eat melons on their own.

4. Do NOT mix acid and/or sub-acid fruits with sweet fruits at the same meal. Acid fruits such as grapefruits, pineapple, and strawberries can be mixed with sub-acid fruits such as apples, grapes, and peaches, but neither of these categories can be mixed with sweet fruits such as bananas, dates, or raisins.

5. Eat only four to six different fruits or vegetables at one meal.

6. Fats and oils combine with everything (except fruits), but should be used in limited amounts because they will slow down digestion.

7. Wait the following lengths of time between meals that don't combine:

   - 2 hours after eating fruit

   - 3 hours after eating starches

   - 4 hours after eating proteins

I've been food combining for years, and along the way I've discovered some of my own personal tips that I want to share with you. These are helpful hints that have worked for me, and they might work well for you too.

For the most part, I divide my day into three food combining segments. I eat fruit in the morning, a protein lunch, and a starch dinner. This gives me a cleansing fruit meal first thing in the morning, my energy-packed protein lunch in the middle of my day, and the slow steady release of energy from eating complex carbohydrates at night. I can't always keep to this routine (especially if my work schedule prohibits it), but I find that it's what really works best for me and my lifestyle. Sometimes I'll eat my protein lunch in the form of a starch-legume (rice and beans, tofu stir-fry, pasta with lentils, or split pea soup with pasta), which makes a complete protein.

If you mis-combine, there are always ways to offset the bad combination. Say you eat a protein with a starch; you can eat some legumes with the starch, and it will "convert" the starch to a complete protein. Let's say you eat chicken with rice for lunch. If you eat some beans (any kind), the chicken-rice combination will digest more easily than if you *don't* eat the beans. If you eat sushi (fish with rice), which is automatically a bad combination, make sure you add either miso soup or edamame (cooked steamed soybeans) to your menu. If beans or soy products aren't available to help round out your mis-combined meals, you can always (in a pinch) eat some peanuts after the meal to offset the bad combination. (Peanuts are fattening, I know, but eating a few will make the digestive process more comfortable and the meal will be less fattening in the long run. This has worked well for me, anyhow.) Speaking of nuts, another good tip is that if you're going to eat a lot of nuts, make sure you eat an acid fruit with them. I had to really figure out this one, because nuts (especially cashews) are one of my favorite indulgences. When I do eat them, I drink a glass of orange juice or eat some other acid fruit. (You can't imagine how many people I've had to explain this little trick to while sitting next to them on an airplane!)

Marilu's Personal Food Combining Tips

1. Divide your day into three food combining segments. Preferably eat fruit only in the morning, a protein lunch, and a starch dinner.

2. Some days you may want to eat your protein lunch as a starch/legume meal, which makes a complete protein.

3. If you experience a 4 o'clock energy slump, try saving some of your lunch to recharge your batteries.

4. If you mis-combine by eating starches with protein, eat some legumes with the starch, and the starch will become a complete protein.

5. I choose not to eat dairy products, but I do eat foods high in calcium so that I get a sufficient amount of it in my diet.

6. Never eat nuts without some acid fruit.

7. If you do eat dairy, combine it with an acid fruit, especially pineapple, which contains bromelain, an enzyme that helps the stomach digest dairy.

8. When drinking alcohol, follow these rules:

   • Drink two glasses of water for every one ounce of liquor, four ounces of wine, or eight ounces of beer.

   • Drink beer and grain alcohol (vodka, scotch, rye whiskey, sake, etc.) when eating starches.

   • Ideally, you should drink wine and champagne only with fruit.

9. Drink spring or bottled water only.

10. Drink liquids 15 minutes before eating or one hour after eating.

Step Seven: Fat

"Fat Free," "Low Fat," and "High Fat" seem to have an overbearing presence in our world these days. People are completely fat obsessed, but it is the type of fat you eat that matters. It's impossible (not to mention unhealthy) to try to maintain a "fat-free" lifestyle. While most people know how much they weigh, very few people know their blood cholesterol level. When I first started my program, it was 237. For the last fifteen years, it has been between 130 and 160. It's an important number to know, because it helps measure your risk for heart disease. A diet high in fat will lead to a higher cholesterol level, making you a candidate for bigger problems later in life. But remember, low fat doesn't mean no fat. Food needs fat to taste good, and quite frankly, our bodies need some fat too.

The Skinny on Fat

Fat in food does do your body some good. It is a necessary nutrient. Fat provides essential fatty acids, from which your body makes molecules it needs to function properly. It acts as a wall of protection around your vital organs like your heart and kidneys. It also acts as an insulator for the body. Fat carries essential (fat-soluble, meaning they dissolve in fat) vitamins A, D, E, and K. These vitamins cannot be absorbed into your body without fat. Although a diet high in fat is unhealthy, fat is the ingredient that makes most foods taste better. Flavor adheres to fat. Fat can offer a concentrated source of energy because fats have a tendency to pack together if they're not in water, so they become a source for greater energy storage. Fat protects your internal organs from going into shock. It insulates the body in extreme temperature conditions. It also acts as an emergency fuel supply in times of illness. Extremely low-fat diets suck the oil right out of your skin. You need a certain amount of fat in your diet for skin to look healthy.

For nutritional purposes, fats can be divided into three categories: saturated, monounsaturated, and polyunsaturated, based on the amount of hydrogen each one carries. *Saturated* fats have no more room for any additional hydrogen. An easy way to remember what a saturated fat is is to think of animals. All animal fats, such as those found in meat, poultry, dairy products, and eggs, are saturated. Chocolate, coconut oil, and products made with lard are also saturated fats. These are considered the least healthy forms of fat because they are the highest in cholesterol. Saturated fats can also cause the body itself to produce higher levels of cholesterol. *Monounsaturated* fats have a little extra room for hydrogen (one more atom) and are somewhat better for you than saturated fats. They are oils like olive, peanut, and canola. Peanut butter and avocados are also monounsaturated fats. People usually think avocados are fattening, but they're not as bad as you think. They're better than eating a saturated fat. *Polyunsaturated* fats have room for many more hydrogen atoms and are the healthiest form of fat. Corn oil is an example of polyunsaturated fat. Fish, soy, corn, sunflower, and safflower oils are all polyunsaturated fats. English walnuts, salad dressings, mayonnaise, and margarine where liquid oil is the first ingredient are also polyunsaturated. Most experts agree that limiting your daily fat intake to less than 30 percent of total calories consumed is the best approach to eating a healthy diet. Interestingly, your daily percent of total calories consumed should not fall below 15 percent from fat. Of course, to stay within this range of 15 to 30 percent, you should try to avoid eating saturated fats as much as you can.

Limiting—Not Eliminating—Fat

Eating too much fat results in some really harmful consequences. The obvious one is that fat makes you fat. Gram for gram, fat delivers more than twice as many calories as carbohydrates and protein. One gram of fat is equal to 9 calories. You have to be really careful with fat-free foods, though, because they tend to be very fattening. Taking the fat out loses the flavor, so food manufacturers compensate by adding other ingredients like artificial flavorings, sugar, and syrups, all of which are high in calories. Read your food labels! Some fats are definitely easier to spot than others are. Butter, cream cheese, salad dressings, mayonnaise, and cheese are all obvious fat foods. Meats like sausage, pepperoni, bologna, bacon, corned beef, and hot dogs aren't as obvious, but they're all high in fat. Ice creams, cole slaw, pasta salads, and potato salad are also high in fat. (Of course, these days, there are a lot of low-fat substitutes for these products.)

Even though fat grams are easier to count, calories are what really do you in. Watching the fat in your diet is important, and balancing your intake between fats, protein, and carbohydrates is the best combination for good health.

Trying to eliminate fat from your diet is hardly the answer to better health. Fat, as I said earlier, is essential to your health. The key is to successfully replace the bad fat with good fat. If you let your fat intake fall below 20 percent calories from fat a day, you may start eating more volume of food because you'll have a harder time getting full. Fats digest really slowly (much slower than carbohydrates and proteins), and they take the longest to exit your body.

Step Eight: Exercise

Dear Marilu,

I am so excited about this whole new way of life! I started an exercise and weight loss program in January and have lost 45 pounds. Since buying your book, I have adopted so many of your steps and they have helped me get off the plateau I was on and continue losing more weight. The difference in how I feel is amazing! I am 32 years old and have never looked or felt better in my life! This was exactly what I needed to jump start me again and really make these needed life-saving changes!!

Debbie Leutza

My final breakthrough in weight loss came once I decided that I would break a sweat for at least 20 minutes every day. I had decided that the gym was too inconvenient and time-consuming and that a personal trainer was way too expensive. All I really needed was to make the time in my schedule to get moving. I would put on a CD, the radio, whatever I could find, and just dance and sweat like crazy. I always felt great after those workouts. I started doing this on December 1, 1987, and by Christmas I had lost 8 pounds! For years, even though I had been eating as well as I did, those stubborn last 10 pounds just wouldn't come off. Breaking a sweat *every day* for at least 20 minutes was the missing piece to the puzzle that I had been trying to solve for years! From that time until now, I have maintained my ideal weight range (except, of course, when I was pregnant) without a struggle. Hallelujah!

I think exercise is so important, I decided to devote an entire chapter to it, so for more information please read Chapter Five.

Step Nine: Sleep

Sleep is the one step in my program that is absolutely essential to helping every other step work effectively. I've never been able to handle a problem, thwart a cold, or solve a beauty drama without a good night's sleep. Sleep is the fountain of youth. If someone told you that you could look younger, feel better, boost your energy level, and keep yourself healthy, wouldn't you want to know how to do that? It's simple, it's cheap, and it's as easy as getting a good night's sleep. Your body has a built-in clock that knows when you are sleep-deprived and when you are right on schedule. You can't cheat your need for sleep without cheating yourself.

Getting enough sleep allows your body to be a natural healer for almost every ailment that can affect you. People who are totally sleep-deprived find themselves down for the count. They literally work themselves into the ground until their bodies give them a reminder to slow down and get essential rest. Sleep is truly one of the greatest gifts you can give yourself. Your body will thank you, your mind will thank you, and everyone in your life will thank you, too—because you won't be crabby! Zzzzz.

Step Ten: Gusto

Dear Marilu,

I have been on your program since Mother's Day, and I have lost 8 pounds already! In the past year I had put on over 25 pounds and all the doctors could tell me is that it was caused by stress. My cholesterol jumped by 30 points over a four-month period. My trainer at the gym said I wasn't eating enough—and now after being on the B.E.S.T plan for over two weeks, I feel great and I believe I am on the road to a healthier me!! Thanks for the great advice.

Laura Hanna
Washington

Gusto has nothing to do with looks. There are many beautiful people who don't have a clue about Gusto. Likewise, someone with Gusto is automatically attractive. Gusto is what separates the people in life who are truly successful and enviable.

Without Gusto, you're merely marking time, and with it, you're devouring time and space. People with Gusto have that look of vibrant health and carry themselves with confidence and self-assuredness. They have that light behind their eyes, and you can't help but find yourself drawn to someone with that kind of magnetism. I'm not saying that you should go through life carefree and with rose-colored glasses on. Life is filled with challenges, changes, surprises, and curves. When we are confused or when we take a wrong turn, we may need some help working through the muddle and getting back on track. It is during these times, especially, that we must believe in ourselves and trust that we can indeed do what we set out to do.

I have found that, in life, attitude is everything. My philosophy has *always* been "The key to your life is how well you deal with plan B." Having resilience—and the ability to get over things and move on—is everything. To be able to ride the roller coaster of life and *still* want to put your hands in the air with joy and excitement every day is the greatest gift to be honored and envied. So many people are afraid of making a mistake that they stay at zero on the number line. They're so afraid of "minus" that they never get to "plus." Sometimes you have to risk being bad (or embarrassing) to get to good. Ask anyone who's taken up a musical instrument, or singing, or dancing. (Or, better yet, ask anyone who has to listen to anyone who's taken up a musical instrument, or singing, or dancing!)

Learning to like yourself is one of the most important steps you can take on your road to health. You do not have to accept living a life where you are uncomfortable with yourself, your body, and your health. You are a work in progress. Change is often the hardest challenge we face in life, but you must not be afraid to face it. Most of us have gotten pretty used to the way we live. We want to change, but we're uncertain how to replace those old habits.

What happens too often is that we become so discouraged with the distance between where we're at and where we want to be that we give up the fight. We make excuses as to why we "can't" change the way things are. Maybe you're too old, too set in your ways, or just too embarrassed to put on a leotard, let alone allow anyone else to see you looking so out of shape. The idea behind Gusto is to break those self-imposed barriers. Guess what? An old dog *can* learn new tricks! Put on that tutu and dance around your house. Break that sweat every day. Build your confidence as you build your health. You must silence that pessimistic voice of self-harassment in your head (that ugly mirror) that holds you back. Becoming aware of that voice is the first step in quieting it down and finally making it go away. If you start to have negative thoughts, so what? We all have them! Have *all* your feelings. Your feelings are not going to kill you. Just use judgment when putting your feelings into action. And remember, accepting who you are and all of your feelings that come with it is Gusto!

You'll always have something that you'll want to change about yourself because as long as you live and breathe, you will remain a work in progress. The ultimate reward in improving yourself is that you will inevitably improve your health and your self-image. Like the rest of my plan, once you take that first step to achieving Gusto and putting faith in a positive attitude, you can't help but graduate to another layer because the changes you're making for yourself are working. You will find that adding Gusto to your life is the "spiciest" ingredient to this new recipe for your life. (Besides, after following this 30-day plan, you will be so organized there will be *plenty* of time for Gusto!)

5

Exercise

I originally wanted to design a 30-day exercise program that would give you some specific routines to develop and follow. I soon realized that exercise is different from all the other components in this program because everyone must approach it in an individual way. What one person finds boring could be pure bliss for another. More important, the ideal exercise program for one person could cause serious injury for another. Even a program designed for beginner, intermediate, and advanced exercisers is not diverse enough to accommodate the wide range of fitness levels out there. I will, however, tell you exactly what my fitness program is as well as give many suggestions so you can create an exercise program that's right for you. To insure proper safety, before you start any exercise program, you should always consult with your physician to assess your fitness level and find your exercise boundaries.

Being a dancer, I always knew that exercise was great for my overall health. I never quite realized until my commitment to break a sweat every day how important it was to do it consistently. The last thing I want is for you to think that exercise is the final step in your makeover program, and that you incorporate it only after you've been able to conquer everything else. In fact, you should think just the opposite. No matter what age or the condition of your health, you should start exercising right away. Remember that safe exercise for one person is completely different from safe exercise for another.

If you're extremely overweight and have been inactive for a long time, exercise for you might be leisurely walking just once around the block or simply sitting in a chair and moving rhythmically to music for five minutes. You're never too old to exercise either, but you must find which exercises are safe and right for *you.*

After all we now know about the benefits of exercise, it is amazing that still only 20 percent of Americans exercise regularly. It is quite clear that exercise reduces stress; lowers blood pressure and cholesterol; controls weight; burns fat; combats osteoporosis; builds, strengthens, and tones muscles; slows the aging process; balances your mood; and simply makes you feel better. Yet 4 out of 5 adults are still not doing it! The reason for this is that many of the 80 percent believe that exercise is not only painful and boring, but that they have to be a certain type of person to do it. This kind of thinking has created a "them and us" schism. It's as if exercise were reserved for Ken and Barbie types with kinesiology degrees. Some non-exercisers feel they have to lose weight, get fit, and learn how to properly use all the equipment before they will even allow themselves to go into a health club. They believe that someday they're finally going to get serious and live their lives right and reap all the benefits that exercise promises. But that day never actually comes.

Why is it that kids don't have the same silly hang-ups when it comes to exercise? It's because kids instinctively do exactly what exercise is all about. They find an activity they enjoy doing, and they do it! Adults have made this issue far too complicated. A good place to start an exercise program is to reclaim the way you thought of exercise when you were a child. It's kind of like learning computers. The reason every kid under 12 knows how to operate a computer, and most adults over 50 don't, is that, unlike kids, they are afraid to simply start "doing it." It reminds me of the Groucho Marx line, "This is so easy, a four-year-old child could understand it. Now run out and find me a four-year-old child. I can't make heads or tails out of it." Exercise should be thought of as "playtime." Isn't it amazing that it's hard to get a child to stop playing and even harder to get an adult to start? Most adults think of exercise as pain, and no one will continue to do anything associated with pain. I'm so glad that ridiculous "no pain no gain" mentality of the '80s is long gone. Children certainly don't associate exercise with pain, and you shouldn't either. I want you to keep this return-to-childhood idea in mind as you create your exercise program. There are hundreds of ways to exercise. Find the ones that you will truly look forward to doing every day.

The five most important components of a successful exercise program are safety, variety, enjoyment, convenience, and effectiveness. Safety is most important for obvious reasons. You can't exercise when you're injured. Variety not only adds spice and keeps you from getting bored; it's important for your body.

"Don't just stick with one type of routine. It is important to vary your workouts. The muscle adapts to the load that is put on it as well as the movement that it's asked to perform. In other words, muscles get bored after a while and don't respond as enthusiastically. Therefore, in order to surprise the muscle and get more force from it, you must vary the resistance, the intensity, and the movement. It's sort of like rotating crops in a field. If a farmer always raises the same crop, the field can become fallow."

Ted Pastrick
Master of Science, Physical Therapy

Your program has to be enjoyable, for all the reasons I mentioned earlier. You have to enjoy something if you have any hope of continuing it for the long term. Remember, find that former child. Also important for the long term is convenience. If it takes a big effort or sacrifice, how long do you think you will continue? Don't sign up for classes in another county. Finally, your routine has to be effective. Movement in itself can be effective, depending on your current fitness condition. Our bodies naturally want to move. If you haven't been moving in quite a while, your body will be grateful for the change, and simple movements will be beneficial. Just like safety, this is very individual. If you're regularly active, you have to do more for your workouts to gain any benefits. Remember that exercise is a building process. Your body gradually strengthens and builds in order to adapt to the workload it faces.

I currently alternate my workouts among my three favorite forms of exercise, which incorporate these three main components:

- **Pilates**—a comprehensive method of exercise that strengthens, stretches, and elongates the muscles while increasing endurance, suppleness, and control. I don't think there's ever been a type of exercise that makes me feel more in balance and more centered. No matter how I am feeling at the beginning of my session, I leave there feeling exhilarated—like I've really done something wonderful for my body. With the growing popularity of the Pilates Method, many Pilates-based variations have sprung up. The best and most correct instructors are certified through the Pilates Studio in New York City. So ask questions.

- **Dancing**—I love to dance, whether it's around my house, in a dance class, or out socially with my friends. It always makes me feel like a kid. I have danced my whole life, and it's life affirming to me. I loved working on Broadway because of all the dancing I got to do. I'm always putting on music and jumping around the house with my kids.

- **Walking or jogging on a treadmill**—This is perfect when I haven't got time for the other two. It's easy, it's fast, and I can catch up on my TV or MTV. It's a mindless way to sweat. I just get on and off within twenty minutes to a half an hour.

These are the things I currently do for my exercise program. I am not suggesting that these would be the best routines for everyone. That is for you to discover. I found them after a long period of trial and error. (Plus, I might change my program in 3 or 4 months to try new things.) The best advice I can give is *Be your own personal trainer.* Pretend that you've hired yourself to assess your fitness goals and design your own personal plan. This will give you an opportunity to step outside yourself and be objective, and it will give you a chance to explore all the options. Learn as much as you can, but don't feel you have to wait to learn too much before you get started. Moving doesn't require a Ph.D.

Here are a few basic tips to keep in mind and help you get started:

1. **All workouts should begin with a brief warm-up and stretch, regardless of what follows.**

2. Decide what your main goals are so you can choose exercises that target your objectives.

3. Resistance training builds muscle tissue, and aerobic training burns fat.

4. Any amount of exercise is beneficial for weight loss. For fat reduction, you should set aside at least thirty minutes for your aerobic workouts, but never reach the point of breathlessness. The body will only start to use its fat reserves after a certain period, and thirty minutes is about the average time when the body switches from burning carbohydrates to burning fat. Fat is a much more concentrated energy source, and the body chooses to burn fat over carbohydrates only after it feels a more intense energy resource is required.

5. If your primary goal is to build muscle mass, use heavier weights with fewer repetitions (6 to 8) for the majority of your workouts. If your primary goal is to tone and sculpt, use lighter weights with more repetitions (12 to 15). To develop endurance, add isometrics to your workout. Don't just stick with one type of routine, though. It is important to vary your workouts.

6. Resistance training done before aerobic training is a more efficient use of your energy than the reverse.

—Ted Pastrick, M.S.P.T.

Choose a fun sport or activity that engages your body in continuous aerobic movement. As stated earlier, aerobic activity needs to be continuous for at least 30 minutes before the body begins to burn fat instead of carbohydrates. Don't, however, be discouraged by this. *Any* kind of safe movement is beneficial to weight control. You can gradually work your way up to 30 minutes or more if you want. *You* have to be your own coach and choose the duration and intensity level. You should never be out of breath (unable to carry on a conversation) or feel any aches and pains. Remember to insert at least a 5-minute stretching routine 3 to 5 minutes into your activity. It's more beneficial to stretch after the body has warmed up a bit. Do some slow movement and static stretching at the *end* of your activity as well.

Beginner: 5 to 15 minutes

Intermediate: 15 to 30 minutes

Advanced: 30 minutes or more

Activity Suggestions

1. Wear a comfortable outfit all day.

Beginner: Don't strain yourself, but keep the words "exercise" and "energetic" in your mind all day. Walk around the block after breakfast. Walk up the stairs. Try not to take any elevators or escalators unless it's a high-rise. Walk around the block again after lunch.

Intermediate: Same as Beginner, plus include the following: a $1/2$-mile walk, 1 minute of stomach crunches, 2 minutes of walking up and down stairs, 10 men's or women's pushups. Do these exercises all at once or spread throughout your day. Make sure you do all exercises slowly and evenly to avoid injury. Slow stretching is always a good idea too.

Advanced: Same as Intermediate, but increase to: 1-mile walk, 3 minutes of crunches, 3 to 5 minutes of stair climbing, and 40 push-ups (4 sets of 10).

2. Find a fun place to walk: the park, the zoo, the mall, etc. Walk without stopping for 20 to 30 minutes. Don't stop at any food courts, hot dog stands, or cafeterias during or after for a reward. Use a Walkman if that adds to the pleasure of your workout.

Beginner: Don't worry about speed. Stroll at a pace that is comfortable and relaxing. Try to make it continuous only if you can. If you get at all tired or out of breath or feel any pain, simply stop.

Intermediate: Walk briskly and continuously for the entire 20 to 30 minutes.

Advanced: Jog continuously for the entire 20 to 30 minutes. Keep your heart rate between 110 and 140 beats per minute, depending on your age and fitness goals.

3. Dance continuously and privately for 30 minutes to your favorite tape or CD. (Remember: This is how Tom Cruise got started.) Have fun and don't exhaust yourself. If you're out of breath from Bob Seger, switch to the Bee Gees. If they tire you out, try Mariah Carey. Still winded? The last resort is Peggy Lee. (If you actually have all four in your record collection, it's time for a garage sale.) Most important of all, make sure the door is *locked*, unless you're hoping for a partner to walk in.

Other suggestions for music:

Beginner: Sarah McLachlin, Sheryl Crow, Van Morrison

Intermediate: *Saturday Night Fever* (sound track)

Advanced: Gypsy Kings, Brian Setzer Orchestra, Big Bad Voodoo Daddy

4. Find a nicely heated pool. Move around comfortably and continuously for 20 minutes in the shallow end. Swimming is one of the best all-around exercises because it offers some resistance along with aerobic training. Best of all, it offers a much lower risk of injury than most other forms of exercise.

Beginner: Move any way you want for the 20 minutes, as long as you don't just sit and simmer like the Jacuzzi people. Also consider a beginner's aqua class.

Intermediate: Do very relaxing, comfortable laps for the entire 20 minutes. Try wading, breaststroke, sidestroke, or whatever is the easiest method you use for simply moving in water. If you get even slightly out of breath, switch to an easier way to move through the water. Also consider an aqua class.

Advanced: Keep an even, brisk pace doing your favorite stroke during the 20 minutes. If you're in great shape but don't know any strokes, try an aqua-aerobics class.

5. Set aside two hours. Put on workout clothes and choose a room that needs organizing. Alternate throughout the two hours between organizing and working out. The

switching keeps you from getting bored. Incorporate loud, energizing music if you like. By the end you'll feel great and have an uncluttered, well-functioning room. Within the two hours you should complete the following:

Beginner:

- 2 minutes of stepping up and down to get warmed up. (March in place if you don't have a brand-name step. Footstools can be dangerous.)
- 5 minutes of stretching
- 1 minute of abdominal crunches
- 1 minute of side leg lifts (½ minute each leg)
- 1 minute inner leg lifts (½ minute each leg)
- 1 minute back leg lifts (½ minute each leg)
- 3 to 10 male or female push-ups (total during 3 sets)

Intermediate:

- 3 minutes of stepping up and down to get warmed up
- 5 minutes of stretching
- 2 minutes of varying abdominal crunches
- 10 to 20 male or female push-ups (total during 3 sets)
- 2 minutes of side leg lifts (1 minute each leg)
- 2 minutes inner leg lifts (1 minute each leg)
- 2 minutes back leg lifts (1 minute each leg)

Advanced:

- 3 minutes of stepping up and down to get warmed up
- 5 minutes of stretching

- 4 minutes of varying abdominal crunches

- 15 to 40 male or female push-ups (total during 3 or 4 sets)

- 2 minutes of side leg lifts (1 minute each leg using a resist-a-band)

- 2 minutes inner leg lifts (1 minute each leg using a resist-a-band)

- 2 minutes back leg lifts (1 minute each leg using a resist-a-band)

6. Shop around to find an exercise video that's perfectly suited for you and work out to it once a week. You'll find an incredible variety these days in levels and interests including country, salsa, Irish, step, and swing. Choose what you really like or want to learn.

The following exercise videos are only meant as a brief guideline. These various instructors tend to guide their workouts toward the following levels.

Beginner: Richard Simmons, Judy Shepard-Misset's Jazzercise

Intermediate: Marilu Henner's Dancerobics, Kathy Smith, Denise Austin

Advanced: "B-Fit" with Tara Phillips and Michael George, Kari Anderson, Karen Voight

I can't stress enough how important exercise is for your overall health.

Exercise is just as important as diet in any health makeover. Make sure you break a sweat *every day*! Your Total Health Makeover will not be as effective if you don't.

6

The 30-Day Program

Countdown

DAY 1

MOTIVATIONAL TIP

CLOTHING CHECK. Take a piece of clothing (jeans, a pair of comfortable slacks, a fitted suit or dress, etc.) that you wear now that fits really well. Either put it aside or keep it in mind, but try not to wear it for the next 30 days. At the end of the program you're going to try it on again to see how differently your clothes fit.

EXERCISE TIP

DON'T MAKE TAKING CARE OF YOURSELF INCONVENIENT. Have all of your exercise equipment and clothes in one area so you don't have to waste the time looking through the rest of your stuff, and you won't have the excuse that you can't find any-thing. I put all of my sneakers, socks, sweats, T-shirts, baseball caps, Walkman, and fanny pack in one convenient spot so that I don't spend twenty minutes rummaging through drawers trying to find something to wear to go out walking. Give yourself all the help you need by conveniently setting yourself up to win.

FOOD TIP

BE CONSCIOUS OF HOW YOU EAT. Do you do unconscious eating? Do you eat in the car? Do you eat standing up? Do you graze at the refrigerator without preparing your-self anything? Do you count that as part of your eating for the day? A lot of times peo-ple are unaware of how much they eat. They pick off other people's plates, or they clean up their children's food before they throw it into the garbage can. Whenever I find myself eating standing up, I know that it's usually out of nervous energy, or because I've waited too long to eat, or because I feel as if I need a reward. It's much better to sit down and have a meal. If you're really going to snack in between, be con-scious of the fact that it is a snack. A lot of times people will buy something to eat in the car. They plan to eat only a little bit of it, and then they'll consume the entire bag. So today, as an exercise, pay attention to how you eat.

ORGANIZATIONAL TIP

SET UP YOUR LIFESTYLE JOURNAL. For the next 30 days, you should not only keep track of what you eat and when, but also the type and duration of any exercise you do and how much you slept the night before. You might want to chart the effects the new foods have on you (gives you energy, liked the flavor, fewer cravings). You can also write down how much you weigh and, if you're a woman, the day of your men-strual cycle. (If you don't want to weigh yourself on this program, you can easily judge your weight loss by how your clothes are fitting.)

The 30-Day Total Health Makeover

BEAUTY TIP

SKIN BRUSH EVERY DAY. Start every morning by using a natural bristle brush. (It can look like a shoe brush or the kind with a long handle, but remove the handle, of course.) You can buy these brushes at your local beauty supply or drugstore. You want to brush your *dry* skin in an elongated upward motion toward the heart for 1 to 2 minutes every morning. Start with your feet and ankles, and work your way up the body to your calves and thighs. Really concentrate on brushing the lymphatic areas of your body (the back of your knees, your inner thighs, and under your arms) to stimulate those glands and get them started on flushing out those toxins. Gently brush up your stomach and tush, shoulders and back. Finish this regime with each arm and hand. Make sure you cover the entire surface of your body, excluding your breasts and face. The brushing should not irritate you. It may take a couple of days to get used to it, but if you hang in there, I promise you will feel the difference in your skin in less than a week.

SPA ON A BUDGET TIP

GIVE YOURSELF AN EGG WHITE FACIAL. I learned this when I was eleven years old (not that I needed to tighten my pores at eleven, but I knew what was coming): 1. Crack open an egg, make sure that the yolk doesn't break. 2. Switch it back and forth between the two half shells, and make sure you get the yolk out of there, so you just have the egg white. 3. Put it on your face, as if you were washing your face with it, and then let it harden. 4. Rinse off with tepid water.

TOTAL HEALTH FAKEOVER

FIND A HEALTH SPONSOR. Tell someone who really has your best interests at heart that you're going to get healthy, and sound excited about it, even if you're not. Their enthusiasm about your feeling better will make you a believer as well. (I can't believe

I'm telling people to lie, and we haven't even gotten started yet.) By telling somebody that really has your best interests at heart, you'll be making a commitment to the next 30 days because you'll feel the encouragement and the love from that person. Just make sure you're not telling someone in your environment that you would *like* to be supportive of you but is *really* a secret saboteur (we all have people like that).

Menu

DAYS 1 TO 4

No formal menu but remember

NO MEAT
NO DAIRY
NO SUGAR
NO ALCOHOL

You should also BREAK A SWEAT (for at least 10 minutes) EVERY DAY while on this program.

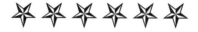

Countdown
DAY 2

MOTIVATIONAL TIP

WRITE DOWN WHAT YOU WANT. As you can tell from this program, I'm somebody who really likes lists and diaries. They not only help keep me organized, but I like looking back on them years later and remembering where I was at that moment. For example, fourteen years ago, after I'd broken up with someone, I decided that I really wanted to fall in love again, and I wanted a great guy. I wrote down in my diary all the qualities that I wanted in somebody. Two months later, I met my husband, Rob. The following year, I was reading that same diary, looking something up, and I saw the list in there. I had forgotten that I had written it at all, but when I realized that it was written on the date of Rob's birthday, I was really amazed! I think it's important to write things down so that they're out in the universe, so it is clear that you are saying, "I really want this in my life." Eventually you'll get it.

EXERCISE TIP

FIT IS MEASURED IN SEVEN WAYS. (Fit doesn't mean skinny.)

1. Endurance

2. Strength

84

3. Flexibility

4. Speed

5. Coordination

6. Agility

7. Equilibrium

Look at these seven ways and assess your ability in each category. You might be more fit than you realize. Hopefully during this program, you will improve in each area. A lot of times people will wait until they look good in a leotard to start moving or working out. I know so many people who say, "Oh, well, I have to lose some weight first, and then I can go to the gym." Forget it. You don't even have to go to a gym. *Ever.* And you *never* have to put on a leotard. Just get moving. Put on comfortable clothes and walk around, jump around, dance around, take a class, do something. Whatever you do, just get your body *moving*! That's how you get fit. You get oxygen in your blood. You get oxygen to your brain. You get that serotonin kicked in. It's very, very important to just keep moving!

FOOD TIP

SIZE DOES MATTER. The important thing to remember with portion size is that you have to listen to your body. I'm not talking about your emotional body, the body that's been created by emotional eating. I'm talking about really letting the signal that you've eaten get to your brain. It takes about 20 minutes to feel full, so make sure that when you sit down to eat, you spend at least 20 minutes. Or get up, move around, go to the bathroom, do one of your organizational tips, whatever it takes, to let it sink in that you've just eaten. You know, so many times we look at a plate of food and we think we have to eat everything that's on the plate. Some of the portions that I'm recommending on this program are going to be too much or too little for you. Even if there's some food left over, that's fine, save it for a snack two hours later or save it for another meal. Start paying attention to how much you eat, not only whether you're eating unconsciously, but also the volume. Let your brain get the signal that your stomach is full.

ORGANIZATIONAL TIP

DON'T PUT OFF TILL TOMORROW WHAT YOU'VE BEEN PUTTING OFF ALL YEAR. Make an appointment for something you haven't done in a long time. Everybody has an appointment that's hanging over their heads. Sometimes it takes weeks to get one, so right now, get up, go to the phone, call your doctor, call your dentist, your gynecologist, your urologist, your pediatrician, whatever. I don't care if you're reading this at two o'clock in the morning, leave a message with their service and make a commitment to set an appointment and then keep it.

BEAUTY TIP

PART OF BEING HEALTHY IS LOOKING NATURAL. The best way to look natural is to put on your makeup in a natural light. Set up your makeup near a window, even if this means you have to use your living room. I learned this the hard way. I used to put on makeup every day in a mirror that had nothing to do with sunlight, and I ended up wearing way too much makeup. Every time I see a photograph of myself from that time, I remember that it was because of the lighting in my apartment that I look like a clown. It's so important for you to put your makeup on in a natural light, *especially* if you work in an office with fluorescent lighting. Make sure you check your makeup in natural light. You'll look a lot healthier as a result.

SPA ON A BUDGET TIP

WASTE NOT, WANT NOT. A "QUARTER" OF SHAMPOO, A "DIME" OF CONDITIONER. I discovered this tip from a hairdresser who was spending so much time trying to get body into my hair, until she finally said to me, "How are you washing and conditioning your hair?" When I told her how much shampoo and conditioner I used, she said, "This is the biggest mistake people make. You really don't need that much shampoo or conditioner." A quarter size of shampoo is sufficient. You don't need to shampoo your hair twice, either. (That recommendation came from when people used to wash their hair twice a week.) When you condition your hair, put a pea size or a dime size in your hands first. Condition the ends of your hair where you need it the most, and then run it through a little bit on the top. People usually glop a huge amount on top of their heads and then spend all their time using products and blow drying to give their hair a lift. Today when you wash your hair, just try using less shampoo and conditioner and see how it works.

TOTAL HEALTH FAKEOVER

MIND OVER MATTER. Have all of your "sick" feelings when you're not feeling well, but don't act on them. As an actress, I've learned that "The show must go on." No matter how you're feeling, you have to do a performance. This is a good trick to do in life as well. Today (or from now on in your life), not everybody has to know what's going on with you all of the time. Sometimes getting yourself through the day by *not* giving in to all of your negative or sick feelings is a much better way to go. Sometimes *acting* like you feel better will help make you *feel* better because you have to do a job and because you have to function. I'm not saying that you have to be a total faker, but sometimes it's better to fake it a little bit to get through your day. Try not to indulge yourself in all of your sick or negative feelings. What you can do is just say, "I'm going to get through this. It's mind over matter."

Countdown
DAY 3

MOTIVATIONAL TIP

THE DAYS DRAG, THE YEARS FLY. Don't let another month go by where you're not at your best. We're on the third day. We're going to be finished four weeks from today. Look at your calendar. What did you do four weeks ago? That doesn't seem like that long ago. After two days on this program you're probably already becoming more conscious of things and the quality of the details in your life are adding up to more than you ever realized. It's just the beginning. If four weeks ago feels like a short time, the next four will go by even more quickly because there's so much going on and you're accomplishing so much.

EXERCISE TIP

TODAY, EVERY TIME YOU'RE AT A STOPLIGHT, DO SOME KIND OF EXERCISE. People usually say they have no time for exercise. How much time do we spend in traffic, either driving or being a passenger? Every time your car is stopped, do something. You can tense the muscles in your arms, squeeze your butt muscles, or tuck in your stomach. Try stretching the back of your neck by rolling your head from side to side in front (make sure you're stopped at the light, of course). Whenever I remember to do this, I feel like I'm getting a little workout in the middle of my day.

FOOD TIP

HOW TO DRINK WITH YOUR MEALS. My rule of thumb is that you don't gulp your drinks with your meals. Drink 6 to 8 glasses of water in between meals, because you want to keep yourself as hydrated as possible. But with your meal, you should just sip whatever liquid you're drinking. What you don't want to do is dilute your digestive juices. Those digestive juices are very specific to the kinds of food that you're eating. If you water them down, they won't work as well. When you chew your food, your mouth sends a signal to your brain to start putting those juices into effect. If you start gulping water, the food passes quickly through your throat, esophagus, stomach, and intestines, and the nutrients aren't going to be pulled from your food. So don't gulp; sip if you're going to drink with your meals.

ORGANIZATIONAL TIP

Never leave a room empty-handed.

—Ingrid Bergman

This is definitely something I picked up from my mother (who probably read it about Ingrid Bergman). I don't think I ever saw my mother leave a room without picking something up. Or, she'd say to one of us, "Here, take these to the kitchen," or "Take this into my bedroom," or "Make sure you get this out of here." It's amazing how much work gets done as a result. Otherwise you're at the end of the day and everything's in the wrong room. If you never leave a room empty-handed, if you make that commitment, things get picked up along the way, and it makes keeping order so much easier. We're talking about streamlining during these 30 days, and this is one of the best ways to do it. It certainly keeps you from having your hands free to pick up food and carry it from the refrigerator into the next room. (Besides, I love the image of Ingrid Bergman working on *Casablanca* and making sure that she carried something from "Rick's Café" to her dressing room.)

BEAUTY TIP

CHECK OUT YOUR CLOTHES IN NATURAL LIGHT. You know how we put on our makeup in natural light? Well, now we're going to check out our clothes in natural light. Take a mirror to a window and put your clothes up to your skin, and see which ones make you look better. What you don't want to do is wear colors that take the coloring out of your skin. I have a couple of colors that look great in my closet, but as soon as I take them into natural light, they "go hospital" on me. (I look like I should be hooked up to an I.V., because they completely drain the color out of my skin.) Also, there are different shades of blacks and navy blues. An outfit that looks great in your closet can look totally different in the sunlight because the shades don't match.

SPA ON A BUDGET TIP

WARM WASH, COOL RINSE. Wash your hair in warm water, and final rinse it in cool water. When you wash it in warm water, your hair shaft opens up, it gets clean, and then you have to make sure you close it up again by giving it a cool rinse. (It's kind of the yin and yang of hair washing.) If you do this, it'll make your hair shinier and more manageable as well. Otherwise you're going to have a lot of frizz and have to use more product, which is going to make it heavy and more difficult to manage.

TOTAL HEALTH FAKEOVER TIP

MIRROR, MIRROR ON THE WALL—PART I. Everyone is influenced by the thin mirror in their house. I know I am. Sometimes I look in my thin mirror, and I think, "Oh man, I really look good today. I'm going to take really good care of myself because I'm on a roll." So today, look at that thin mirror and walk, talk, and dress like the "thin" person you see (even if you don't feel like you're there yet). Just look at yourself and say, "I'm really looking good, and just think, I'm going to look even better."

Countdown
DAY 4

MOTIVATIONAL TIP

EVERYTHING IS CONNECTED TO EVERYTHING. I'm sure that while you're reading this book, there are things that I've said in the first couple of chapters that you're already relating to the rest of your life. It's like when you're a child and you learn a new word and then it seems like the whole world is using it. That happens as an adult, too. It's really important to make certain connections in your life and to be sure that you're paying attention and relating things. You'll start to feel more in control of your life because you'll no longer feel like you're in a vacuum and all the forces around you are manipulating you one way or another. You'll start making connections in your relationships to people, as well. One of the important things I hope to accomplish on this program is to have people relate the way they live to the way they eat.

EXERCISE TIP

IDENTIFY YOUR EXERCISE PERSONALITY. Are you a *social* exercise personality? Somebody who likes aerobic classes, gym, hiking clubs, group interaction, dance classes, anything where you're with a lot of other people and you're doing things together? Not so much in a competitive way, but rather, there are a lot of different people in the room. Are you an *intimate* personality? Somebody who likes to exercise one-on-one, or with a work-out buddy or a trainer? There's just the two of you, somebody who's helping you, somebody who's doing it with you. You like the interaction of having that social time with one other person and so part of your conversation becomes part of your workout. Are you a *competitive* exerciser? Sports teams, racket sports, marathons, team sports, anything where you're competing against another person, or there's a team of people competing against another team? Are you a *solitary* kind of person, the person who works out to a fitness video or does yoga? You focus inward, and participate in something where it's extremely personal. Or are you a *networker*? Do you use exercise for an opportunity to meet career-boosting people? You go beyond the natural athlete in you and the person who's trying to get healthy and exercise, and you see it as an opportunity to make connections. Spend the day figuring out what kind of exerciser you are, and it will help you choose what kinds of exercises you want to do over the next four weeks.

FOOD TIP

GET TO KNOW CONCENTRATED FOOD. A concentrated food is your protein or your starch, around which you can build your meal. What vegetables, what salads, and what else do you put with it? The important thing to remember is that you shouldn't have too many concentrated foods at one meal, and ideally you should only have one *type* of concentrated food per meal. Also, make sure that there's at least one food on your plate that doesn't have oil or margarine or any kind of fat on it. Make sure there's a steamed vegetable or a little bit of salad that doesn't have something that's coating it in some way. That wet food will definitely help you to digest the concentrated food.

ORGANIZATIONAL TIP

GET RID OF ALL FOOD SABOTEURS. Go through your cupboards and get rid of anything that may ruin Boot Camp. You don't have to throw it out (although it's probably better if you do). Just put it somewhere so you won't be able to see it, so you won't feel like "Oh my gosh, there's my favorite food." Put it in your freezer, but don't eat it. Out of sight, out of mind. Don't feel as if you have to have it around for your husband or your kids. They shouldn't be eating unhealthy food, either. If you have to keep it around for them, make sure it's someplace that you're not going to automatically go to, especially when no one's looking. If somebody in your environment is the saboteur, then put them in the freezer as well.

BEAUTY TIP

MAKE FRIENDS WITH YOUR NAKED FACE. Spend the whole day without makeup or take off your makeup as soon as you're home for the night. You'll spend less time clogging your pores with heavy, hours-old makeup, and you'll be sure to clean your face well instead of being too tired and doing a feeble job late at night. As an actress, I love the days that I don't have to wear makeup because I feel like my skin is getting a vacation. It can breathe. So many people are afraid to go around without makeup, but I think people actually look better *without* makeup. It's so nice to walk around and have your natural face.

SPA ON A BUDGET TIP

ICE, ICE, BABY! After you've washed your face and before you use toner or moisturizer, rub an ice cube all over your face to tighten up your pores. (Men can do this, too!) It's amazing what will happen. It's cheap. It's effective. It's the same thing we did with our hair the other day. A cool rinse closes up the hair shaft. An ice cube on your face tightens up your pores. (Don't be ashamed, guys, because it's really a great trick!)

TOTAL HEALTH FAKEOVER

WAKE UP 15 MINUTES EARLIER THAN YOU NORMALLY DO. Start your day collecting yourself before your schedule begins so that the moment you wake up you're not in overdrive. You will end up doing things more efficiently throughout the day if you give yourself that extra time. Fifteen minutes is not very long, but for some reason, it feels more like an hour when you use that 15 minutes first thing in the morning. It's not going to make that much difference in your sleep, but it'll kick start you in a way that you won't feel like you're playing catch-up all day long. Tomorrow we're going to start Purple Week. So starting tomorrow, wake up 15 minutes earlier.

During the next 26 days, you will be given menus for breakfast, lunch, and dinner. If at any time the food is not available to you, the following substitutions are permitted. I've also included a list of 7 approved "on the go" meals.

1. For a protein meal, you can substitute 6 to 8 ounces of grilled, broiled, or poached fish. Make sure it is prepared with as little oil or margarine as possible. (No butter, of course!) You can have a side order of steamed vegetables and a salad with no more than 1 tablespoon of all-natural non-dairy dressing.

2. For a starch meal, you can substitute any type of pasta with a non-dairy, non-meat tomato sauce. In a restaurant, ask your server to make sure the sauce is a plain tomato sauce. Serve with a side order of steamed vegetables and a small salad with no more than 1 tablespoon of all-natural non-dairy dressing. Or, you can substitute steamed brown rice and vegetables. Serve with a small salad with no more than 1 tablespoon of all-natural non-dairy dressing.

3. For a grain-legume meal (which makes a complete protein), you can substitute the protein meal listed above (#1) or simply add tofu to the steamed brown rice and vegetable combination listed in #2.

4. If there's a particular meal that you really like within one week's menus, you can repeat that meal or save your leftovers for another meal. Make sure you stay within each week's color. No substituting a "Yellow Week" meal in "Boot Camp." It's best if you only substitute a protein meal with a protein meal and a starch meal with a starch meal.

5. If for any reason you find that it's easier for you to swap your lunch and dinner meals, go ahead and do that.

7 "ON THE GO" MEALS

1. A scoop of tuna salad on a bed of lettuce. No extra dressing!

2. Angel hair pasta with tomato sauce (no dairy, extra light oil.)

3. Salad Niçoise, with no potatoes and no egg yolks. No more than 1 tablespoon of all-natural non-dairy dressing.

4. Vegetarian non-dairy soup with a whole-grain roll.

5. Vegetarian cheeseless pizza.

6. Grilled or broiled fish (no butter, light oil) with steamed vegetables.

7. Vegetable stir-fry.

Please note: At any time in this program, you may eat fruit only (see page 61 for proper combinations) in place of a starch or protein breakfast.

Boot Camp

DAY 5

PURPLE WEEK KITCHEN LIST

Everything you will need for Purple Week's menus

Check your kitchen for what you already have. Check recipes for amounts.

Vegetables
Arugula
Broccoli
Cabbage, red or green
Carrots
Celery
Cucumbers
Garlic, fresh
Green beans, fresh
Green beans, frozen
Mixed greens
Onions: white, red, yellow
Peas, frozen
Plum tomatoes
Scallions
Spinach

Tomatoes, vine ripened
Zucchini

Herbs & Spices
Basil, fresh
Cumin
Dill, fresh
Italian parsley
Oregano, fresh
Paprika
Parsley, fresh
Tarragon

Fruits & Juices
Apples
Cantaloupe

Carrot juice
Grapes
Honeydew
Juices of choice
Oranges
Pineapple
Seasonal fruit

Grains, Breads, Pasta
Brown rice
Cereal (Puffins, Shredded
    Spoonfuls, Oatios, etc.)
Flourless whole grain bread
Oatmeal
Rye

96

Protein

Ahi tuna

Eggs

Salmon

Swordfish steaks

Tuna, canned in water

Miscellaneous

Balsamic vinegar

Bragg's Liquid Aminos

Burdock root tea

Capers

Chamomile tea

Dijon mustard

Extra virgin olive oil

Maple syrup

Miso

Nayonaise

Parchment paper

Peppermint tea

Red clover tea

Red wine vinegar

Relish

Rice Dream

Soy margarine

Vegetable concentrate or stock

MOTIVATIONAL TIP

**Listen to what you say.
You may mean it.**

—James L. Brooks

We spend years of our lives talking about the changes we want to make . . . someday. How many times have we said, "I'm really going to get in shape one of these days," or "At some point, I'm going to get my act together," or "I'd really be able to stick to a plan if I just knew what to do." Well, that day, that someday, that one of these days, is today. If you're really serious about what you've been saying, if you really mean it, you can do it. You just have to put your mind to it.

EXERCISE TIP

PLAY CLOTHES ALL DAY. Try to spend as much of the day as you can wearing sneakers and workout clothes to feel like you want to move all day. You'll burn a lot more calories moving around than trying to look taller by wearing uncomfortable high heels. When I was on *Taxi*, I always thought I'd look long and lean by wearing tall boots. If you watch, you'll see that in almost every *Taxi* episode I have on these stupid boots. (It's amazing I never developed any back problems.) When I think about all the times I wore boots to rehearsal and in the show, when I could have been more comfortable, moving more efficiently, and burning more calories, I could kick myself with those boots!

FOOD TIP

BACK TO THE GARDEN. The first thing we're going to bite into is a nice, juicy apple. I feel like it's biblical in a way. It's metaphorical. It's what took Adam and Eve out of the Garden of Eden, but it's going to put you right back in. It's the start of this program. You're going to spend this morning really tasting that apple. It's one of the first things I really started to taste again. I bit into an apple years ago, and I tasted the flavors, and I want you to do that, too. (Hopefully you've gotten an organic one, because the flavor is better.) How many times have we bitten into an apple and eaten it, but not really tasted it? We're trying to retrain our palate and really taste foods again. This is how it starts. (If there's not a lot of flavor to things today, you might need a few more days before you really start to taste your food.)

ORGANIZATIONAL TIP

I SEE LONDON, I SEE FRANCE. Check out your underwear. Get rid of any that are stretched out or don't fit (unless they're a goal size), or are just too ugly for even your ugly days. Try it on or size it up by just eyeballing it. Take the whole pile of it with you when you watch television tonight. It should take you about fifteen minutes to do the whole thing. Remember, your mother always told you . . .

BEAUTY TIP

NOW YOU SEE IT, NOW YOU DON'T. A yellow concealer will help even out red skin tones (red patches on your cheek or a pimple). A peach concealer will help even out blue skin tones (dark circles under your eyes or veins). Sometimes you have to use a little of both in the same spot. This is a trick I learned years ago when I ended up on the cover of *Redbook* with not one stitch of makeup on my face and a so-called beauty picture right next to it. (This was in the mid-eighties, so I hadn't gotten my act together yet, and you could see the residual effects of dairy and sugar still on my face.) They took a yellow concealer and put it on all the red parts of my face. Anything that was splotchy or where I had a pimple. Then they put peach concealer on anything around my eyes or wherever there was any darkness. I've used this makeup trick ever since.

SPA ON A BUDGET TIP

PEOPLE, PEOPLE WHO NEED PEOPLE. Use olive oil on your fingernails and cuticles as a conditioner and moisturizer. I got this tip from the world's greatest manicurist and pedicurist. Shelley does everyone that you've ever seen in *People* magazine with great nails, so you know she's very good at what she does. She says to use just a dot of oil on each finger or toe, to keep nails healthy.

TOTAL HEALTH FAKEOVER

I'D RATHER BE BLUE. Wear a color that makes you look healthier. For example, match the color of your eyes or find the right color of blue that makes your skin look vibrant. Newscasters and talk show hosts often stand in front of a blue background because it brings out their skin tones. This is also why people on television usually look so healthy. The right blue is a great fakeover color.

Menu

DAY 5

Breakfast: 1 apple, 1 orange, and 1 cup of grapes to be eaten throughout the morning until two hours before lunch

Mid-morning: Chamomile (for tranquility), peppermint (for digestion), red clover (for energy), or burdock root tea (for weight loss)

Lunch: Donna's Vegetable Soup with 1 cup rice and rye combination (see recipes to follow)

Snack: A handful of raw green veggies: broccoli, cucumbers, green beans; and/or peppermint, red clover, burdock root, or chamomile tea; and/or carrot juice

Dinner: Salad 101 with Dressing 101, Salmon in Parchment, 2 cups steamed broccoli

> Remember, during Boot Camp it's important not to feel like you're starving. If you get hungry, try a glass of water. If that doesn't do it, have a cup of Donna's Vegetable Soup (without the rice and rye).

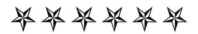

Pot of Rice and Rye — Lunch

SERVES 4

This is one of the first dishes I learned to make when I decided to get healthy. Someone told me that rye literally sucks the fat out of you, and I believe them.

- **4 cups water**
- **1 cup brown rice**
- **1 cup rye**

Bring water to a boil. Add rice and rye. Bring to boil and simmer until liquid is absorbed. Throughout Boot Camp, you will be adding rice and rye to soups and other dishes.

Donna's Vegetable Soup — Lunch

SERVES 8

Donna Erickson has been our nanny and surrogate grandmother since the day our son Nicky was born. She's one of the world's greatest cooks, and her soup always makes us feel lean and healthy. You will be using it again in Boot Camp.

- **2 tablespoons vegetable concentrate (Organic Gourmet Instant Soup N. Stock, or any healthy vegetable concentrate)**
- **1 onion, chopped**
- **2 tablespoons chopped parsley**
- **2 cups chopped celery**

2 cups chopped carrots

2 cups zucchini, cut into chunks

2 cups cabbage

2 cups frozen green beans

Add vegetable concentrate to 2½ quarts hot water, or adjust amount of water to taste. Add onion, parsley, celery, carrots, and zucchini and cook soup on low heat for 10 to 15 minutes. Last, add cabbage and frozen green beans. Continue cooking on low heat about 5 minutes. Never overcook vegetables.

JoAnn's Salmon in Parchment—Dinner

SERVES 1

JoAnn Carney, my oldest sister, is a successful photographer and the best cook in the family. Her dishes are fast, easy, and look as good as they taste.

Parchment paper (found in store near aluminum foil)

6 to 8 ounces salmon

1 teaspoon olive oil

Dill to taste

⅛ teaspoon black pepper

1 teaspoon chopped scallions

Preheat the oven to 375 degrees. Tear off a piece of parchment paper so that it makes a square. Fold it in half so you have a triangle. Open the paper and place the fish on the inside crease. Sprinkle the fish with olive oil, a little dill, black pepper, and scallions to taste. Fold the top of the paper over. At the side, begin taking tiny little folds overlapping on top of the other, sealing the contents inside tightly. (It will look like a turnover.) Bake for 12 minutes or more to the doneness you prefer.

Salad 101 and Dressing 101 — Dinner

SERVES 1

1 teaspoon olive oil
1 teaspoon balsamic vinegar or white or red wine vinegar
1 teaspoon Dijon mustard
2 cups mixed greens
½ tomato, sliced
½ cucumber, sliced

In a small bowl, combine olive oil, vinegar, and mustard and mix well. Drizzle on top of the salad and toss.

Boot Camp
DAY 6
PURPLE WEEK

MOTIVATIONAL TIP

FIND A "GOAL" PIECE OF CLOTHING. Either find it in your own closet (a favorite old dress, a pre-pregnancy outfit, an old pair of jeans) or buy something you would love to wear in a realistic future size. Hang it in your closet as inspiration. Check your progress from week to week until it fits or almost fits. Years ago, before I left for Spain to do a movie, a friend of mine gave me a pair of pants that were too small, but I brought them with me anyway. I was determined that someday I would wear them, and sure enough, through diet and exercise, by the time I finished the movie, two months later, they fit me perfectly. I still have them and try them on from time to time just to be sure they still fit!

EXERCISE TIP

TAKE A WALK! The trick to staying with an exercise program is to keep it simple and make it fun. What could be more convenient than a brisk walk around your neighborhood? While walking, there are certain images that might help you. Try not to walk hunched over. Posture is very important. One of the greatest ways to remember the proper way to walk is to think of helium balloons holding up your head, your shoulders, and your chest, helping move you forward. Don't look at the ground, but walk and look above the horizon. Otherwise your whole posture will be dragged down. If you look above the horizon, you're going to be moving well and your body is going to end up at about a five-degree angle, the best angle for walking. If you swing your arms, you're going to get even more of a workout. I remember hearing a story that Rose Kennedy used to swing her arms when she walked, and that's probably why she lived to be over 100.

FOOD TIP

A LITTLE DAB'LL DO YA! Dilute salad dressing with a little bit of water and apply it with a small spray bottle. Or try using your fork to drizzle dressing over your salad instead of heaping it on with a spoon. Throughout this program, we're going to be finding ways to cut back on fat and calories. This tip works for gravy or sauces too. Another great way is to put a capful of dressing in a bag (like a salad bag), and then put the salad in, blow a little air into it, and shake it up. This way the entire salad gets tossed, but you've used a very limited amount of dressing.

ORGANIZATIONAL TIP

SOCK IT AWAY! Yesterday it was underpants. Today it's socks! Organize your sock drawer. Get rid of mis-matched socks or socks that have holes in them. Bring the whole load of them in front of the TV or stand there (it should take you about five or ten minutes). Anything that's been sitting there as a single, toss out or make a puppet out of it for your kids. If you don't have the time today to organize your sock drawer because you have too many socks, then make it a point the next time you put the laundry away to do it in an organized way. Eventually all the stuff that you use all the time will be organized.

BEAUTY TIP

DAY 6

PURPLE

ONLY YOUR HAIRDRESSER KNOWS FOR SURE. When shopping for a new shampoo, if your hair is blond, look for a blue-based shampoo to make it brighter. If your hair is brown, find a brown-based shampoo, and for red hair, a red-based shampoo. I learned this shampoo trick from my good friend and hairdresser for years, MaryAnn Hennings. Most of the time I have red hair. But for the different roles I've played, the color of my hair determines the color of my shampoo. You can find these colored shampoos at drugstores or at salons. When I don't do this tip, my hair does not look as vibrant.

SPA ON A BUDGET TIP

CONDITION(ER) YOUR LEGS. If you want really silky smooth legs, try shaving with hair conditioner instead of shaving cream. This works well even with a semi-dull blade, so be careful when using a new blade. I discovered this by accident one day when I ran out of shaving cream. I was actually using a blade that wasn't brand new, and it worked even better than it did with the women's shaving creams that I was buying. I've been a devotee of this tip ever since then. I feel like I've saved myself a lot of money as well because you don't need a lot of it. Just put a thin layer of conditioner on your legs, and shave your way to the smoothest legs ever.

TOTAL HEALTH FAKEOVER

THE SHAPE OF THINGS TO COME. Even if you're not the size you want to be, you can still show your shape. Find some part of your figure to show off. Are you a tight top and baggy bottom person or a tight bottom and baggy top person? Big, baggy clothes tend to make people look bigger than they are. They also scream out to the world, "I'm trying to hide!" There's always something that can look more shapely and smaller as a result of a better fit.

Menu

DAY 6

Breakfast: ½ of a melon, cantaloupe or honeydew (or ¼ of each), or 1 cup pineapple

Mid-morning: Chamomile, peppermint, red clover, or burdock root tea

Lunch: Salad Niçoise

Snack: A handful of raw green veggies: broccoli, cucumber, string beans; and/or chamomile, peppermint, red clover, or burdock root tea; or carrot juice

Dinner: Confetti Rice and Rye

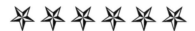

Salaд Niçoise — Luncb

SERVES 1

Mixed greens

1 tomato, chopped

Handful green beans, raw or steamed

2 hard-boiled egg whites, optional

6 ounces grilled ahi tuna or 1 six-ounce can of tuna packed in water, not oil

Dreϑϑing

1 tablespoon olive oil

1 teaspoon balsamic vinegar or white or red wine vinegar

1 teaspoon Dijon mustard

On a bed of mixed greens, place the chopped tomato, green beans, and hard-boiled egg whites. Season the tuna steak with a little bit of salt and pepper. Cook on a hot, clean grill about 3 minutes per side (inside should be bright pink). Place the grilled or canned tuna in the center of the salad. In a small bowl, combine the olive oil, vinegar, and mustard and mix well. Drizzle the dressing over entire salad.

Confetti Rice and Rye—Dinner

SERVES 3 TO 4

¼ **cup vegetable broth**

¼ **cup minced red onion**

¼ **cup chopped celery**

½ **cup julienned red cabbage**

½ **cup frozen peas**

2 **cups cooked brown rice and rye combination (see page 101 for recipe)**

⅛ **cup chopped fresh parsley**

⅛ **cup chopped fresh basil**

In a large saucepan, combine the vegetable broth, red onion, celery, cabbage, and peas. Bring to a simmer. Add rice and rye combination, parsley, and basil. Heat at low temperature for an additional 3 to 5 minutes.

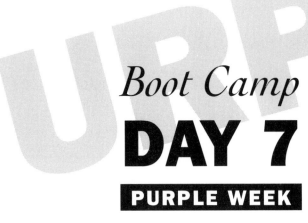

Boot Camp
DAY 7
PURPLE WEEK

MOTIVATIONAL TIP

The problem is the solution disguised.

—Dick Guttman, publicist

This is one of my favorite tips of the entire program. Most people don't realize that you can take every problem and twist the perspective on it to find the solution within it. I do this at least once a day. For example, my weight problem was my health solution disguised. If I hadn't spent years being overweight, having bad skin, and suffering the emotional consequences, I would never have been inspired to find a healthier way of life.

EXERCISE TIP

BEND ME, SHAPE ME. All day, think of yourself as an athlete. I don't care what you do, I don't care what size you are. You move in your own life, so start becoming aware of motions you do every day that simulate exercises. Free weights mimic what we do in real life. When you reach for something, really reach for it. When you lift something, use your legs, use your stomach muscles. Pick it up. Pick up those groceries. Pick up those kids. It's amazing how much more you'll get out of your day.

FOOD TIP

YOUR STOMACH DOESN'T HAVE TEETH. You're trying different foods. Maybe you're eating grains for the first time in a long time. Make sure you chew your food. Unless you chew every single bite, you're not going to lose weight, you're not going to get the nutrients, you're not going to have a clean colon, you're not going to digest properly. You're eating vegetables, you're eating things with fiber. Make sure you chew. The ideal is fifty chews per bite, but aim for at least thirty. (Not that you have to be obsessed with counting it, of course, but chew your food more than those eight bites that you usually do.)

ORGANIZATIONAL TIP

GIVE YOURSELF A LIFT. Okay, ladies, we're going to check out our bras. You should do this at least twice a year. Get rid of any that are stretched out. You could size them up, hold them up, see which ones have the backs all stretched out, and get rid of them. There's nothing worse than a bad bra that's not doing its job. Also, a lot of people walk around with a bra on which the straps haven't been pulled up, so everything is pulling them forward, and it's affecting their posture. Make sure that the back of the bra is pulled down and the straps are pulled up, and it'll give you a lift. You'll look thinner and better right away and be more supported. I'm sure the guys are still working on their socks from yesterday's tip (they usually have a lot more socks than we do). So keep at it, guys! We're going to tackle our bras today.

BEAUTY TIP

FACE IT. Cleanse and moisturize your neck and chest as part of your face regimen. The neck is one of the first places to show age, so you have to take care of it. Until a facialist told me this a few years ago, I only washed and moisturized my face. Now I include my neck, chest, and décolletage.

111

SPA ON A BUDGET TIP

DAY 7

PURPLE

TAKE YOUR MOISTURIZER FURTHER. Put it on immediately after you wash your face. If you use a toner, apply it first and then apply your moisturizer right away. That will keep the moisture on your skin that's left over from your shower or from washing your face. The whole idea of putting on any kind of moisturizer on our face is to keep it on the skin. Otherwise it's just putting something on top of dry skin, and it doesn't really seep in.

TOTAL HEALTH FAKEOVER

BAG BUSTERS! One of the biggest things that makes us look unhealthy is circles under the eyes. A lot of times it comes from weak kidneys, menstrual problems, smoking, or too much sugar. It also comes from a lack of sleep, not enough water, or just plain old exhaustion. (You could be getting sleep and still be exhausted.) A great way to "fake it" is to keep two tablespoons in the freezer, and as soon as you wake up in the morning, or throughout the day, you can put those two tablespoons (the back of them) right under your eyes. This contracts and tightens the skin underneath your eyes. You can also make chamomile tea ice cubes. Brew a pot of chamomile tea. Put the tea in an ice cube tray and make ice cubes out of it. When you need to energize your eyes, take out one of those ice cubes and put it on the skin around your eyes. It's very effective.

Menu

DAY 7

On Rising: 6 ounces of fruit juice or 1 piece of seasonal fruit

Breakfast: (2 hours after fruit) 1 piece flourless whole-grain bread with ½ pat soy margarine

Mid-morning: Chamomile, peppermint, red clover, or burdock root tea

Lunch: Donna's Vegetable Soup with Brown Rice and Rye left over from Day 5 (see page 101). 1 cup soup and 1 cup rice and rye.

Snack: 1 or 2 handfuls of raw veggies: broccoli, cucumbers, green beans, strings beans, and/or carrots; and/or peppermint, chamomile, red clover, or burdock root tea

Dinner: Bragg's and Olive Oil Swordfish with Arugula and Grilled Vegetable Salad

Bragg's and Olive Oil Swordfish — Dinner

SERVES 1

1 6- to 8-ounce swordfish steak
1 tablespoon olive oil
1 tablespoon Bragg's Liquid Aminos

Poke the swordfish with a fork. Whisk the olive oil and Bragg's together. Coat the fish with the oil mixture on both sides so that it seeps into the holes. Grill or broil about 4 to 6 minutes on each side to desired doneness.

Arugula and Grilled Vegetable Salad — Dinner

SERVES 4

2 tablespoons balsamic vinegar
¼ teaspoon Dijon mustard
1 teaspoon water
1½ teaspoons mellow barley miso
1 tablespoon olive oil
Pepper to taste
1 medium-sized sweet onion, peeled and cut into thick slices
1 medium zucchini, cut diagonally into ¼-inch slices
4 to 6 cups torn or coarsely chopped arugula
2 tablespoons whole basil leaves
1 tablespoon chopped Italian parsley

Whisk together the vinegar, mustard, water, and miso. Dribble in the olive oil, whisking constantly until dressing emulsifies. Season with pepper to taste. Brush the onion and zucchini with dressing and grill or broil, turning once, until tender. (If the zucchini slices are particularly large, cut in half lengthwise after grilling.) Toss together the arugula and basil leaves with just enough dressing to coat. Divide among 4 salad plates. Arrange the grilled vegetables on top and sprinkle parsley over all.

Boot Camp
DAY 8
PURPLE WEEK

MOTIVATIONAL TIP

Age is something that doesn't matter unless you are a cheese.

—Billy Burke (a.k.a. Glinda the Good Witch)

**Cheese is something that doesn't matter
because you're on this program.**

—Marilu Henner (a.k.a. the B.E.S.T. Witch!)

Forget about age (and cheese)! **YOU'RE NEVER TOO OLD TO GET HEALTHY AND TO FEEL BETTER THAN YOU DO RIGHT NOW.** A person only feels old if they feel they're not where they want to be, and they don't have the time to get there. But that's not any of us!

EXERCISE TIP

WHEN TO WORK OUT. For me, the best time to work out is first thing in the morning. It really gets my metabolism kick started for the whole day and gets me moving. However, a lot of people can't work out first thing in the morning, and they're really evening exercisers. The best time to do it is *whenever you'll do it*. Just figure out what kind of person you are and how it fits into your schedule. It's doing it that counts.

FOOD TIP

IF YOU EAT BEFORE YOU EXERCISE, YOU SHOULD EAT SOMETHING LIGHT. It's best to have some kind of food at least a few hours before you exercise, whether it's a piece of toast or a bowl of oatmeal. I only eat fruit before I exercise, but that's what works for me. (My husband is the opposite. He can't eat anything, especially fruit.) Figure out what works for you. Water should never be ice cold when you drink it during exercising. It should really be room temperature or only slightly cooler. Freezing cold water is just going to contract everything and give you "brain freeze."

ORGANIZATIONAL TIP

A TISKET, A TASKET, CLEAN OUT YOUR DIRTY BASKET. It's important to make a good presentation when you're trying to get healthy. Clean out and organize your purse, wallet, briefcase, and/or tote bag. Throw out those shredded tissues, stale gum, receipts, coupons, flyers, and any old food! (Think of all the loose change you're going to find, too!) Your bag or purse is your portable living space. If it looks organized, you'll look organized.

BEAUTY TIP

SHOULD YOU WEAR MAKEUP WHEN YOU EXERCISE? That's up to you. A lot of times people don't want to go to the gym not looking good because it's become a social thing. (Here in Los Angeles especially, the person working out next to you could be your next boss.) If putting on a little makeup is going to make you work out better because you're going to have to look at yourself in a mirror, then by all means, put on a little makeup. If you're working out at home, do whatever you need to do to get yourself through it. It's really whatever you want. It is much better to let your skin breathe, so make sure you *don't* put on a really heavy base. A light, tinted moisturizer is better.

DAY 8

PURPLE

SPA ON A BUDGET TIP

FIRST AID KIT IN A BOTTLE. Next time you're in a health food store, get a product called tea tree oil. I call it a first aid kit in a bottle. It's an all-purpose first aid solution for burns, cuts, scrapes, rashes, pimples, infections, earaches, and cold sores, and it's a great insect repellent as well. It's an antifungal, antibiotic oil, with antiseptic abilities. My kids find it especially healing, and it's not expensive. It's amazing because you use just a drop of it, and it's extremely effective. It takes the place of so many products you usually have to buy.

TOTAL HEALTH FAKEOVER

REACH OUT AND TOUCH SOMEONE. First thing in the morning, call someone who will put you in a good mood for the rest of your day. For me this is always calling my sister Christal. She lives in New York, so if I wake up early on the West Coast, I can call her because I know she's up. No matter what's going on in our lives, she always puts me in a good mood. She has a very therapeutic effect on me. I could be hassled, I could be stressed. But when I talk to Christal it just reminds me of what a loving sister I have and all is right with the world. There is someone special like that in your life, so call that person.

Menu

DAY 8

On Rising: 6 ounces of fruit juice or 1 piece of seasonal fruit

Breakfast: (2 hours after fruit) Nicky's Favorite Oatmeal

Mid-morning: Chamomile, peppermint, red clover, or burdock root tea

Lunch: Tuna Salad

Snack: Two handfuls of raw veggies: broccoli, cucumbers, green beans, string beans, and/or carrots; and/or peppermint, red clover, chamomile, or burdock root tea

Dinner: Fiesta Brown Rice

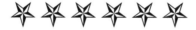

DAY 8

PURPLE

Nicky's Favorite Oatmeal—Breakfast

SERVES 1

Nicky is my four-year-old son, and he loves to eat oatmeal. It's simple to make and really good for you.

> ½ cup oatmeal (quick)
> ¾ cup boiling water
> ½ teaspoon maple syrup

Put the oatmeal in a bowl, add the boiling water, and drizzle with maple syrup.

Tuna Salad—Lunch

SERVES 1

> 6½-ounce can tuna, water packed, drained
> 1½ tablespoons Nayonaise
> 1 tablespoon Dijon mustard
> 2 cups mixed greens

Optional items to taste

> **Relish**
> **Onions**
> **Dill**
> **Celery**

Mix all the ingredients in a bowl and enjoy.

Fiesta Brown Rice — Dinner

SERVES 4

¼ cup diced carrots

¼ cup diced white onions

1 teaspoon minced fresh garlic

1 cup diced zucchini

1 large red plum tomato, diced

1 tablespoon olive oil

½ teaspoon paprika

¼ teaspoon cumin, optional

1 tablespoon fresh oregano or ½ teaspoon dry oregano

1 cup brown rice

2½ cups water

Sauté all the vegetables in olive oil. Add the seasonings and stir in the brown rice. Sauté for another 3 to 5 minutes. Add the water, turn the heat to high, and boil all the water out. When all the water is gone, lower the heat to the lowest setting, place the lid on, and leave for 15 to 20 minutes. No peeking or stirring!

Boot Camp

DAY 9

PURPLE WEEK

MOTIVATIONAL TIP

TAKE CARE OF YOURSELF THE WAY YOU WOULD YOUR BABY OR CHILD. If you're feeling like you want to give up and go back to your old habits, treat yourself as you would your child. This tip was inspired by one of my best friends, Caroline Aaron, who is a brilliant and funny actress. She always says that when she does this, it just sets up her day. She has a beautiful baby girl, Sydney, and whenever she really wants to take care of herself, she imagines that she's like Sydney. She wouldn't give Sydney a cup of coffee and a cigarette. If you feel like blowing it today because you're frustrated, or you're thinking you're just going to do Boot Camp and go back to your old ways tomorrow, just think about how you would want to take care of someone you really love. You have their best interests at heart, and you want to see them be the best version of themselves.

EXERCISE TIP

HAPPY FEET! I discovered from my podiatrist that you should put a thin coat of Vaseline on your feet and wear two pairs of socks for your workout. It's amazing how it not only saves your feet from a lot of wear and tear and scaly skin, but also it makes your workout so much easier. You're not getting bumps, and you're not getting blisters. My husband does it, too. He runs every day, and it has really saved his feet as well.

FOOD TIP

BE PREPARED! Surround yourself with healthy food choices. Next time you go shopping, don't buy those unhealthy things that you usually stock your refrigerator with. Don't make it so difficult on yourself, especially in the beginning. Get the healthy choices so you won't be tempted.

ORGANIZATIONAL TIP

START A REPLACEMENT LIST. Keep a pencil and tablet handy in your bathroom, bedroom, or any other convenient place. Jot down all the things you need to replace. We've cleaned out our sock drawer, bra drawer, and underwear drawer. Some of those things may need to be updated. If you keep a list, next time you go shopping you'll see it listed and know at a glance what you need.

BEAUTY TIP

STUCK IN A RUT? Try wearing a different lipstick, a new hairstyle, or a different perfume or cologne. You can always go back to your old ways, but for one day rethink an old habit. You know, we're trying to think of our lives in a different way, our eating habits in a different way. Maybe there's something new you've been dying to try. (For you guys, maybe you want to grow a mustache or shave one off.) If it's too drastic, don't do it. But if you feel like you've been stuck in a rut for a while, and the new you is starting to emerge, maybe you should experiment with one little thing today and see if it has an effect. I'm always trying this with lipsticks. (Sometimes it works, and sometimes it doesn't.) If you want to try this tip when you're home by yourself just to see how you look in the mirror all day, that's fine, too. It's really good to update yourself once in a while, and this is a fun, easy way to do it.

SPA ON A BUDGET TIP

B.E.S.T. FOOT FORWARD. If your feet are dry and flaky, coat them in Vaseline. Put on a clean pair of cotton socks, and sleep with the socks on. This is especially good after wearing sandals. This is a cheap way to get your feet soft. (I like wearing socks to bed. I always did, I guess, because I grew up in Chicago, and it was freezing cold. I do this tip a lot.)

TOTAL HEALTH FAKEOVER TIP

DON'T STOP THINKING ABOUT TOMORROW. Tonight, see if you can either lay out your clothes or set the table for breakfast or do something else that takes time in the morning. I grew up in a small house, with six kids, eight people, and one bathroom. My mother always had us lay out our clothes the night before, and it made morning time a little less crazy and made us feel less stressed starting our day. It's still something that I do as an adult. I do it for my kids, I do it for myself, and it just makes me feel like I'm more on top of things.

Menu

DAY 9

On Rising: 6 ounces of fruit juice or 1 piece of seasonal fruit

Breakfast: (2 hours after fruit) ¾ cup cereal with ½ cup Rice Dream (Puffins, Shredded Spoonfuls, Oatios, etc.—any healthy cereal without refined sugar or chemicals)

Mid-morning: Chamomile, peppermint, red clover, or burdock root tea

Lunch: Fiesta Brown Rice (leftovers from dinner, Day 8; see recipe, page 121)

Snack: 2 handfuls of raw veggies: broccoli, cucumber, green beans, string beans, and/or carrots; and/or peppermint, red clover, chamomile, or burdock root tea

Dinner: Elena's 15-Minute Salmon with Steamed Spinach

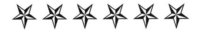

Elena's 15-Minute Salmon — Dinner

SERVES 1

Elena Lewis is a good friend who cooks fast, easy dishes. If she can make this, you can make it too.

> 1 teaspoon red wine vinegar
> 1 teaspoon olive oil
> 1 teaspoon capers or less to taste
> 1 teaspoon fresh parsley
> 1 medium-sized salmon steak (6 to 8 ounces)
> 1 cup steamed spinach

Whisk the vinegar and oil together. Add the capers, then the parsley. Pour the mixture over the fish. Wrap in tinfoil and bake at 400 degrees for 10 to 15 minutes, or until firm to the touch. Place on top of the steamed spinach.

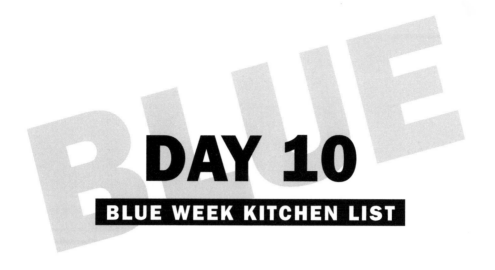

DAY 10

BLUE WEEK KITCHEN LIST

Everything you will need for Blue Week's menus

Check your kitchen for what you already have. Check recipes for amounts.

Vegetables
Artichoke hearts, canned
Bell peppers: red, yellow
Broccoli
Cabbage, red or green
Carrots
Cauliflower
Cucumbers
Fennel
Garlic, fresh
Ginger
Green beans, fresh
Mixed greens
Mushrooms: portobello,
    shiitake, white
Onions: white, red, yellow,
    scallions
Peas, frozen
Plum tomatoes

Scallions
Shallots
Vine-ripened tomatoes
Zucchini

Grains, Breads, Pasta
Brown rice
Bulgur
Cereal
Cornmeal
Flourless whole grain bread
Fusilli pasta
Oatmeal
Pasta shells
Whole wheat pastry flour

Protein
Eggs
Salmon fillet

Sea bass
Shrimp
Striped bass
Sushi-grade Ahi tuna

Herbs & Spices
Baking powder
Basil, fresh
Cilantro, fresh
Cinnamon
Crushed red pepper flakes
Dried basil
Dried oregano
Fennel seeds
Ginger
Ground white pepper
Marjoram
Mint, fresh
Oregano, fresh

Paprika
Parsley, fresh
Poppy seeds
Rosemary, fresh
Saffron
Sage, fresh
Sesame seeds
Thyme, fresh
Vanilla extract

Fruits & Juices
Carrot juice
Grapes
Juices of choice
Lemon
Lime
Pineapple

Seasonal fruit
Spicy tomato juice
Strawberries

Miscellaneous
Arame (seaweed)
Balsamic vinaigrette
    dressing
Chamomile tea
Corn oil
Daikon (seaweed)
Dijon mustard
Honey
Light soy sauce
Maple syrup
Mirin
Miso

Olive oil
Olive oil spray
Peppermint tea
Pickled ginger
Red clover tea
Red wine vinegar
Rice Dream
Rice vinegar
Soy cheese
Soy margarine
Soy sauce
Stone-ground mustard
Sun-dried tomatoes
Tahini
Tamari
Toasted sesame oil

Okay, here we are at day ten, the beginning of the rest of our lives. You've been through Boot Camp. Now it's time to incorporate some other things, a little less strict, and you'll start eating the way I eat all the time.

MOTIVATIONAL TIP

YOU LIVE UP TO YOUR TOYS. This comes from a story that involves my husband. Years ago when he first moved to Los Angeles to get into the film business, he was living in a tiny, depressing apartment with no furniture. He felt as if he would become a loser if he stayed there, so he decided to go out on a limb and kind of hedge his bet on his future. He went and got a place that was not out of his price range, but just a nicer apartment that made him feel more successful. While Rob was hammering nails into the wall the first night, the guy from downstairs came up and knocked on the door. Rob got nervous, assuming the guy was going to complain about the noise. Instead, he said, "I heard somebody pounding and was hoping to borrow some tools." They started talking. The guy turned out to be a film editor and invited Rob to observe him at work. Eventually Rob also became an editor and later a very successful film director. Since that time, his philosophy has been "If you surround yourself with an environment that makes you feel successful, eventually you will be successful." *You live up to your toys.* The toys I'm talking about are healthy food, a good attitude, and organized space. I'm *not* talking about going into debt!

EXERCISE TIP

REDISCOVER THE CHILD IN YOU. No one had to force you to go out and play when you were a kid. Nobody had to force you to go and work up a sweat. Recapture some of that childhood magic by doing something that you used to do as a child. Just go out and sweat and think of yourself as that sweaty little kid who had to be called in for supper and screamed and cried because you didn't want the playing to end. Think of your exercise today as playtime. And if you're really good, your mother might let you stay up late.

FOOD TIP

USE FLAVORED SPRAY OILS TO COAT A PAN INSTEAD OF HEAPING ON GLOBS OF OILS AND MARGARINES. There are so many great flavored oils available, and you can find them in any grocery store. You're going to end up using a lot less fat by just lightly spraying your pan. If you can't find a spray, put a little bit of oil and move it around with a paper towel or your fingers. (Come on, I know all cooks use their fingers.) The flavored oils will also help give a little punch to whatever it is that you're cooking. You won't end up using a lot of salt or other spices that will make you crave sweets. (Don't forget that it's all about balance.)

ORGANIZATIONAL TIP

START A FAMILY CALENDAR. Many of us have appointment books, and a lot of times we live with other people who have appointment books. Sometimes wires get crossed. The way we've handled it in my family is to have a large family calendar in our kitchen. Everybody writes their appointments on it so we all know what we're doing at all times. This is especially great with children because you won't double-book or miss important events. Your spouse won't have one agenda with friends, and the kids and you won't have a different one.

BEAUTY TIP

MAKE TIME FOR BEAUTY. Don't make yourself last on your list of things to do. Find pockets of time to take care of yourself throughout your day. Most of us can do two things at once. (Sometimes you can even do three at once!) Give yourself a manicure while you're on the phone. Take off your makeup while listening to messages. I think it's important not to wait until you're so exhausted that you don't do anything for yourself. Better yet, double-team some of the responsibilities with your husband or your roommate.

SPA ON A BUDGET TIP

SHOP IN YOUR OWN CLOSET! I love this tip. I do it as often as possible. I used to think of my suits and clothes as one outfit, but they're really two separate pieces. Double your wardrobe. Break up your suits. Wear a dressy jacket with jeans. Have a little flair when you dress. Mix vintage with contemporary or velvet with another kind of texture. You can definitely mix and match styles. Wear a tailored jacket with a long, straight skirt, or a T-shirt with velvet pants or skirt. You can even mix decades if you're really daring. If you have the style flash card, go for it. It's amazing how when you open your mind to it, there are so many things in your closet that you never realized had any potential. As my brother Tommy always says, "The charm is in the mix."

TOTAL HEALTH FAKEOVER

GET READY, 'CAUSE HERE I COME. Nothing fakes your mood better than the right music. As an actress, I'm always using music to help put me in whatever emotional state I need for my character. A friend of mine who is a salesman blasts rock music in his car to pump him up before a presentation. Even my four-year-old likes to listen to the Temptations' "Get Ready" when he dresses for school. Find the music that puts you in a winning mood and a productive mood.

Menu

DAY 10

On Rising: 6 ounces of fruit juice or 1 piece of seasonal fruit

Breakfast: (2 hours after fruit) Joey's French Toast

Mid-morning: Chamomile, peppermint, red clover, or burdock root tea

Lunch: Bel's Alive Pasta Salad

Snack: 2 handfuls of raw veggies: broccoli, cucumber, green beans, and/or carrots; and/or peppermint, red clover, chamomile, or burdock root tea

Dinner: Steamed Sea Bass with Scallions and Ginger with Dancing with Ginger Side Dish

Joey's French Toast — Breakfast

SERVES 1

Joey is my three-year-old son, and this is one of his favorite recipes!

1 egg white with splash of rice milk
Dash vanilla extract
Dash cinnamon
1 slice flourless, whole grain bread

Combine the egg white, rice milk, vanilla, and cinnamon in a bowl. Whisk well. Dip the bread into the liquid, coating well, and cook on a nonstick griddle or pan lightly greased with soy margarine.

Bel's Alive Pasta Salad — Lunch

SERVES 4

Isabel Williams (a.k.a. Bel) is a friend of our family's who can make the best foods out of the fewest ingredients.

1 pound fusilli pasta, cooked
1 head broccoli
1 large carrot, thinly julienned
1 zucchini, julienned
2 red plum tomatoes, seeded and julienned
1 cucumber, seeded and diced

½ medium red onion, quartered and thinly sliced
¼ cup low-fat, non-dairy, all natural dressing of your choice. You can also use my recipe for Dressing 101 on page 103.

Cook the pasta until *al dente* and set aside. Thinly slice the whole head of broccoli into small pieces. In a large bowl, toss all the ingredients together and add the dressing.

Steamed Sea Bass with Scallions and Ginger — Dinner

SERVES 4

1 2-pound sea bass fillet
¼ cup sweet rice vinegar
¼ cup light soy sauce
1 tablespoon rice syrup
1½ cloves garlic, minced
1½-inch piece of ginger root, peeled and shredded
6 scallions, shredded

Place the fish, skin side up, on a heat-proof serving plate. Combine the vinegar, soy sauce, rice syrup, garlic, and ginger and pour it over the fish. Turn the fillet several times to coat thoroughly with this marinade and set aside for 20 minutes.

Sprinkle the scallions over and around the fish and place the plate on a steamer rack over rapidly boiling water. Cover tightly and steam until the fish is white throughout and flakes easily. Allow 10 minutes cooking time for each inch of the fish's thickness at the thickest point of the fillet. Remove from the steamer.

Dancing with Ginger Side Dish — Dinner

SERVES 4

4 dried shiitake mushrooms

1 head broccoli

¼ pound fresh mushrooms

½ cup diced carrots

3 tablespoons toasted sesame seeds

¼ cup pickled ginger

¼ cup tahini

2 teaspoons tamari

Soak the shiitake mushrooms in hot water for 30 minutes. Drain and squeeze dry, then slice. Cut the broccoli into florets and steam with the shiitakes until tender. Refresh under cold water and transfer to a mixing bowl. Add the fresh mushrooms, carrots, and sesame seeds and toss. Drain 3 tablespoons of juice from the ginger into a small bowl. Mince the ginger and add to the bowl with the tahini and tamari. Pour over the vegetables and toss.

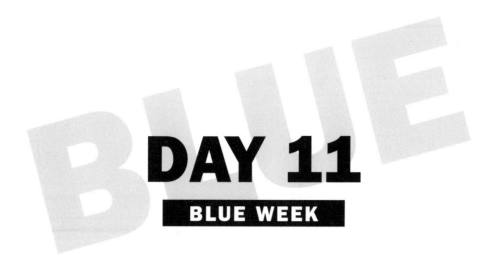

DAY 11

BLUE WEEK

MOTIVATIONAL TIP

PICTURE YOURSELF THIN. Take a photo of your face and tape it to a picture of an outfit that would fit the ideal version of your shape. Most of us know what will look good on us, or at least what we would *like* to look good on us. Usually you take a picture out of a magazine and say, "Oh, I want to wear that someday." If you put a picture of *your* face on that outfit, then you can actually visualize yourself looking great in it. It's kind of fun and silly, but it works!

EXERCISE TIP

POSTURE DAY. We all know that standing up straight will make you look five pounds thinner. You should visualize an imaginary line down the center of your body being pulled taut. Check yourself throughout the day. When you get in the car in the morning, sit up straight and adjust the mirror. At the end of the day, if you can't see yourself in the mirror, don't readjust the mirror. Readjust your posture. If you're used to carrying your purse on one side and your shoulders pull down on that one side, switch your purse to the other side. If you can't switch sides because you're just too used to it, put the strap over on the other side, across your body, and that'll balance you better. If you're used to carrying your kids on one side, carry them on the other side. Just be conscious of correcting your posture today.

FOOD TIP

QUICK DIP. Plunge foods into boiling water quickly whenever possible rather than starting them off in cold water. This avoids oxidation and preserves vitamins A and C. This is why blanched vegetables taste better, retain their color, and are so much better for you.

ORGANIZATIONAL TIP

DAY 11

BLUE

WHEN IN DOUBT, THROW IT OUT! Today, the women are going to go through our makeup drawers and bags, and the guys are going to go through their toiletries. What we're going to do is sort through and get rid of anything that's old. If it smells rancid, throw it out. Mascara should never be more than three to six months old. (Your eyes are very sensitive.) Take those old lipsticks and either try them on or put them up next to your skin tone in natural light. Don't rely on fluorescent office lighting, which is too blue, or household lighting, which is too yellow. I'm sure everybody's got that shoe box of old makeup. After evaluating your makeup in natural light, either keep it for yourself or put it in another shoe box (you're going to give it to your friends later on). Men, it's the same thing. Go through that counter of all those toiletries, all those different shampoos. Go through the things that you don't use all the time and put them aside for friends.

BEAUTY TIP

FILL IN YOUR FLAWS. Whenever I sit in a makeup chair, I always tell the makeup artist that I have a couple of flaws on my face that we have to watch out for. (I've even nicknamed them.) I like to fill in those flaws before applying makeup so that I'm starting with a clean canvas. (It's like spackling a wall before you paint it.) The little things under my eyes are called the "dents" and the little mole I have on my neck is called the "bites" (because it looks like Dracula bit me). Any lines on the side of my mouth I call the "puppets," and my frown lines are called the "horns." Have a sense of humor about your flaws, and learn how to fill them in. One of the greatest makeup "erasers" I've discovered is a peach pencil by Arbonne International.

SPA ON A BUDGET TIP

GOING, GOING, NOT GONE. While we're cleaning out our makeup drawers, help your makeup go a lot further. Foundation bottles are often shaped in such a way to make you have to buy a lot more, a lot sooner. If you add some moisturizer with sunscreen to your foundation, you'll end up with a tinted moisturizer. It's really nice on a light day, or if you're going to work out and want a little makeup to even out your skin tones. Sometimes your pencils have a waxy buildup. The best way to get rid of that is to sharpen them first, and if they still seem hard, put them up to a lightbulb for a few seconds. Don't let them melt completely, just soften the wax. I said before that mascara should be thrown out if it's old, but lipsticks can be scraped with the tip of a Q-Tip, and they're usually as good as new.

TOTAL HEALTH FAKEOVER

PUT ON A HAPPY FACE. Make up your face to look healthier. Think about the way a child's face gets flushed when they run around a lot. Put your blush not so much on the cheekbones (in that dramatic cheekbone area), but more in the apples of your cheeks. Maybe a little bit higher than you normally would. Make sure it's blended, blended, blended so that it doesn't look like blush at all. If you're not the blush type, put on bronzer all over your face as though you've got a suntan. (Some people have a golden look to their skin, other people like a pinky look.) For your eyes, create a more wide-eyed, open look by making sure that you curl your eyelashes and put on your mascara in an upward direction. For lips, dab on a color closest to your natural lip color or just use a dot of clear gloss in the center. There are so many ways to make yourself look healthy and not painted. People will notice.

Menu

DAY 11

On Rising: 6 ounces of fruit juice or 1 piece of seasonal fruit

Breakfast: (2 hours after rising) 1 or 2 pieces of flourless whole-grain toast with ½ pat of soy margarine on each

Mid-morning: Chamomile, peppermint, red clover, or burdock root tea

Lunch: Hot to Trot Tabouleh

Snack: 2 handfuls of raw veggies: broccoli, cucumber, green beans, and/or carrots; and/or peppermint, red clover, chamomile, or burdock root tea

Dinner: Sweet 'n' Easy Grilled Tuna with Steamed Broccoli

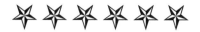

Hot to Trot Tabouleh — Lunch

SERVES 4

1 cup bulgur
¼ cup frozen peas
¼ cup chopped mint
4 scallions, minced
½ cucumber, seeded and diced
1¾ cups spicy tomato juice

Place the bulgur in a strainer and rinse with cold water. Transfer to a Thermos. Add the remaining ingredients, except the juice. Heat the juice to a boil. Pour it into the Thermos and stir to combine. Seal the Thermos lid and let stand for 2 to 8 hours, shaking the Thermos occasionally to mix the salad.

Sweet 'n' Easy Grilled Tuna with Steamed Broccoli — Dinner

SERVES 1

1 small shallot, minced
¼ cup vegetable broth
1 tablespoon balsamic vinegar
6 to 8 ounces Ahi tuna

In a glass bowl, combine the shallot, vegetable broth, and balsamic vinegar. Poke holes in the tuna with a fork (both sides). Let marinate for 20 to 30 minutes. Grill or broil 3 to 5 minutes on each side. Serve with 2 cups steamed broccoli.

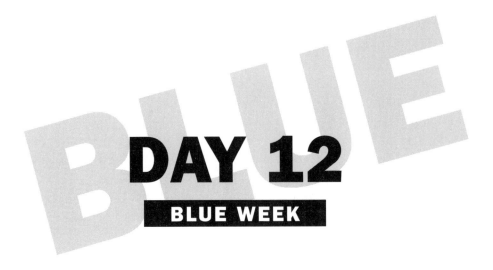

DAY 12

BLUE WEEK

MOTIVATIONAL TIP

FORTUNE, WHO GIVES AND TAKES AWAY ALL OTHER HUMAN BLESSINGS, HAS NO POWER OVER COURAGE. So, if you are not blessed with a great metabolism, delicate ankles, or perky breasts, you can still have the courage to be the B.E.S.T. and the healthiest you. You can't blame bad luck; you must rely on courage in order to be the best you can be. There is no real overnight success, but there is success. Ninety-nine percent of the time, success is based on experience, hard work, knowledge, and timing. The harder you work, the luckier you get. (*Healthy Healing*)

EXERCISE TIP

SINGING IN THE PAIN. Try walking while listening to one of your favorite musicals. One of the easiest ways to work out, if you can afford it, is to walk at home on a treadmill that faces your TV and VCR. Put on a tape of your favorite movie musical and run during the musical numbers and walk during the dialogue, even if it is only for 20 minutes at a time. This is something I discovered years ago when the movie *A Chorus Line* was on television. If sad movies do it for you, shed pounds while you shed tears watching *Casablanca*.

FOOD TIP

TAKE A CALCIUM SUPPLEMENT. I take a calcium-magnesium supplement every single day: 1,000 mg of calcium and 500 mg of magnesium. This was recommended to me by my doctor years ago. (He also told me that it was a natural diuretic, which cleans out your kidneys and keeps everything moving freely.) Make sure that you get calcium citrate, because that's the one that goes directly to your bones. It should also be in the calcium-magnesium combination and with some vitamin D. You need them at the same time so that the calcium gets absorbed. People always assume that because I don't eat dairy, I'm not getting enough calcium from my food. I get plenty of calcium from eating a lot of salmon, soy products, and green vegetables (all on this diet). Women need to get extra calcium, and calcium-magnesium is the best way to make sure you're getting it.

DAY 12

BLUE

ORGANIZATIONAL TIP

CLEAN UP THAT MAKEUP DRAWER AND EVERYTHING THAT GOES IN IT. Wipe off the tops and sharpen the pencils. If it's all over your counter, just keep organizing it until you have it in shape. Wherever you keep it, wipe it clean. Get little boxes that fit into your drawers if you have to. Let's get organized with our makeup so it's not just one big messy drawer that you're just throwing things into. You can always take a rubber band and put it around the pencils, or get some kind of envelope for your brushes.

BEAUTY TIP

FIVE STEPS AND OUT THE DOOR. You should be able to put on your makeup in five steps in the morning. For me, my five steps are concealer, blush, eyebrows and lash line (with the same color and brush), mascara, and lipstick, and out the door. It takes me less than three minutes. Certainly for events or for stage I wear more, but this is just my natural makeup look, and it doesn't take that long.

SPA ON A BUDGET TIP

CLEAN YOUR BRUSHES WITH SHAMPOO. It's unnecessary to spend all that money on expensive brush cleaners. Some brush cleaners can cost ten dollars for a very small bottle. All you need to use is a little shampoo diluted with water. Don't use one that detoxifies or one that is for color-treated hair. Just a mild shampoo or a baby shampoo and soapy water, and that'll clean your brushes. Some makeup artists even recommend using conditioner as well. Just be sure to reshape and air dry.

TOTAL HEALTH FAKEOVER

GIVE YOURSELF SOMETHING TO LOOK FORWARD TO OR TO FEEL OBLIGATED TO LOOK YOUR BEST. Fake yourself out by setting an important date or meeting as a goal to take better care of yourself. Sometimes if you think you've got an important date or an important appointment, job interview, photo session, or special event (a high school reunion or something like that), you get ready for it. Either pretend that you have one or set one in the not-too-distant future.

DAY 12

BLUE

Menu

DAY 12

On Rising: 6 ounces of fruit juice or 1 piece of seasonal fruit

Breakfast: (2 hours after fruit) ¾ cup cereal with ½ cup Rice Dream (any healthy cereal without sugar or chemicals)

Mid-morning: Chamomile, peppermint, red clover, or burdock root tea

Lunch: Portobello Burger Dijonay

Snack: 2 handfuls of raw veggies and/or a cup of the usual teas

Dinner: Salad 102 with Dressing 102, Healthy Miso Salmon with Green Beans

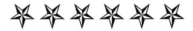

Portobello Burger Dijonay — Lunch

SERVES 1

1 portobello mushroom cap
1 teaspoon Nayonaise
¼ teaspoon Dijon mustard
½ teaspoon capers

DAY 12

BLUE

Gently clean the portobello cap with a damp cloth. Grill the cap approximately 3 minutes on each side. Mix the Nayonaise, mustard, and caper to make the Dijonay sauce. Serve on a whole grain bun with lettuce, tomato, and Dijonay sauce.

Salad 102 with Dressing 102 — Dinner

SERVES 2

4 cups mixed greens
½ cucumber, sliced
3 scallions, chopped
¼ cup broken broccoli florets
1 tablespoon olive oil
1 teaspoon balsamic vinegar
½ teaspoon soy sauce

Combine all the ingredients and serve.

Healthy Miso Salmon — Dinner

SERVES 2

½ cup miso
3 tablespoons mirin (Japanese liquid seasoning)
2 tablespoons minced fresh ginger
2 8-ounce salmon steaks (look for the leanest pieces)
1 cup steamed green beans

DAY 12

BLUE

Mix the miso, mirin, and ginger. Coat the sides of the salmon pieces with the miso mixture. Set in a ceramic or glass pan and cover with tinfoil. Let stand at room temperature for 1 hour. Scrape the marinade from the salmon steaks. Grill or broil the salmon over medium-high heat 5 to 6 minutes per side. Serve with green beans.

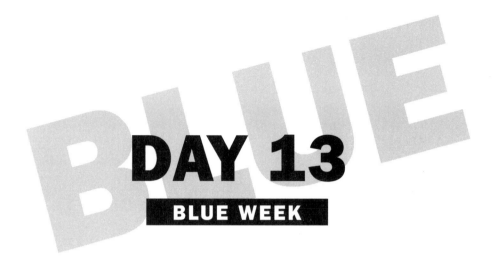

DAY 13

BLUE WEEK

MOTIVATIONAL TIP

IT'S NOT JUST GUT FILL ANYMORE. Food is not your enemy, but a powerful friend. Just respect its properties. Have a good time with it. You're paying attention to your food a lot more than you did before. Maybe you're saying, "Oh my gosh, I had no idea, I didn't even know what miso was." Just respect the fact that food isn't working against you but rather working for you. Dine when you eat. Sit down, really enjoy it. It's not just gut fill anymore. That's your mantra for the day. It's not just gut fill anymore.

EXERCISE TIP

GET A NATURAL HIGH! Drug of choice: endorphins. A lot of us used to drug ourselves with food. Now we're going to turn our attention to a different kind of drug. It's the high that you get from endorphins by taking care of yourself and working out. I like to think of it as having your body *and* your brain sweat. It's putting oxygen in your blood, and that's what's going to make you feel so much better. If you have allergy problems, you're going to be able to breathe a lot better. It's just getting everything moving. Besides, once you get "addicted" to being healthy, you can't stop yourself. That's a healthy addiction—an addiction to making yourself your best.

FOOD TIP

GIVE UP YOUR MEMBERSHIP IN THE "CLEAN PLATE CLUB." We're starting to get more food now. Maybe you're cooking your food, and somebody else in the house is eating something different. Just don't taste their food. Don't pick at what's on their plate. Don't do the Mommy Syndrome, and don't eat while you cook. You're really on a program here, and it's important that the food combinations work for you.

ORGANIZATIONAL TIP

GOOD THINGS COME IN SMALL PACKAGES. Fill a mini-sized bag of your makeup essentials for your everyday purse. How many times do you put on your makeup in the morning, and then decide that you have to take your lipstick or blush to work? I know this might cost a little extra money to get started, but it's such a good idea because you'll eventually use all of the makeup anyway. I have this little satellite bag, and it saves me at least 5 minutes in the morning by not having to sort through my regular makeup bag. After a week, hey, I've saved 35 minutes!

DAY 13

BLUE

BEAUTY TIP

AVOID THE RAGGEDY ANN LOOK. When I was working on the movie *Man on the Moon*, starring Jim Carrey, one of the makeup artists taught me that after I put on my blush, I could easily warm up the tone of my whole face. Take the blush brush that you've been using, making sure there isn't a whole wad of blush on it, and dip it in your powder. Then put it all over your face. That's how you powder over your blush and balance out the rest of your face. This gives your face a nice warm glow.

SPA ON A BUDGET TIP

KITCHEN SCRUBS. If you want to make a scrub with a product that you have at home, you could use oatmeal, which has a nice texture to it. You can also try a wheat germ scrub, which is very, very light. You don't have to spend a lot of money on facial scrubs. If you use a cleansing gel, you could always add a little bit of wheat germ or oatmeal to that, and it'll turn your cleansing gel into a scrub.

TOTAL HEALTH FAKEOVER

DAY 13

BLUE

SEE YOUR TRUE COLORS. What are your power colors, and what are the colors that help your mood? What are the colors that you like around you? I know you have already checked out your clothes in natural light, but think of the colors in your environment more in terms of the items you have around your house (your furniture, your wall coverings, etc.). I'm not saying refurnish the house. I'm not saying recover every single sofa or pillow. Just know that the colors you have chosen are going to have an effect on you.

Menu

DAY 13

On Rising: 6 ounces of fruit juice or 1 piece of seasonal fruit

Breakfast: (2 hours after fruit) Nicky's Favorite Oatmeal

Lunch: Lorne's Blackened Ahi Tuna Salad

Snack: 2 handfuls of raw veggies and/or the usual teas

Dinner: Cleopatra Salad (Caesar Without the Fat), Danny DeVito's Tomato-Mint Pasta

Nicky's Favorite Oatmeal—Breakfast

SERVES 1

½ cup oatmeal (quick)
¾ cup boiling water
½ teaspoon maple syrup

Put the oatmeal in a bowl, add the boiling water, and drizzle with maple syrup.

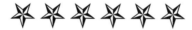

Lorne's Blackened Ahi Tuna Salad—Lunch

SERVES 1

My stepson, Lorne, is a fabulous cook like his dad, and this is one of my favorite dishes he makes.

6 to 8 ounces fresh Ahi tuna (sushi grade)
Dijon mustard
½ teaspoon poppy seeds
¼ teaspoon crushed black pepper

DAY 13

BLUE

Cut the raw tuna into 1-inch-by-1-inch strips. Rub the strips with Dijon mustard. Have a plate prepared with a mix of poppy seeds and black pepper. Roll the Dijon-rubbed tuna with the poppy/pepper mix to cover the fish completely. Lightly wrap the tuna in aluminum foil. Heat the skillet on medium-high. Place the tuna in aluminum in the skillet. Heat for 1½ minutes, turn over, and heat 2 minutes. Remove from heat and place in the freezer for 10 to 20 minutes (cooling the fish makes it possible to cut thinner slices).

To serve, remove the tuna from the foil. Slice on a diagonal with a very sharp knife. Place over the salad pre-tossed with salad dressing.

Salad

2 cups mixed greens
1 plum tomato, chopped

Dressing

1 tablespoon basil olive oil

1 teaspoon Dijon mustard

1 teaspoon red wine vinegar

A sprinkle of poppy seeds

Fresh ground black pepper

Combine all the ingredients in a small bowl and mix well.

DAY 13

BLUE

Cleopatra Salad (Caesar Without the Fat) — Dinner

SERVES 4

1½ pounds freshly mixed greens (organic preferred)

¼ cup minced parsley

2 tablespoons light miso

2 tablespoons water

1½ tablespoons Dijon mustard

1 clove garlic, minced

Soy Parmesan-style cheese, optional

Clean and dry the greens. In a large salad bowl, combine the greens and parsley. Cover with a clean kitchen towel and chill until just before serving. In a small mixing bowl, combine the miso, water, mustard, lemon juice, and garlic. Whisk well to blend. Just before serving, drizzle the dressing over the salad and toss. Sprinkle with soy Parmesan if desired.

Danny DeVito's
Tomato-Mint Pasta — Dinner

SERVES 4 TO 6

Danny DeVito is one of my favorite people in the whole world, and he is an incredible cook. Here's one of his easiest and tastiest recipes.

DAY 13

BLUE

2 tablespoons olive oil
2 to 3 cloves garlic
Mint (big bunch), washed and stemmed
4 plum tomatoes, blanched, peeled, and chopped
1 pound medium-sized pasta shells
Salt and pepper

Make a paste of the olive oil, garlic, mint, and tomatoes using a mortar and pestle. Cook the shells al dente, drain well, and cool. Toss the tomato-mint mixture with the shells. Add salt and pepper to taste.

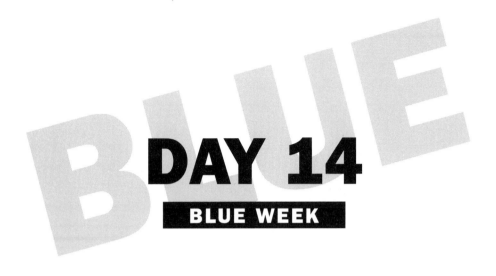

DAY 14

BLUE WEEK

MOTIVATIONAL TIP

With proper care, the human body will last a lifetime.

—Rudolph Ganz, composer

BREAK THE MOLD OF AGING. What kind of lifetime are we talking about? It has to be about quality as well as quantity. Aging, for the most part, has a lot to do with how we treat ourselves. The human body is designed to last between 110 and 120 years. Middle age should mean 60! Our mothers put on 10 pounds at 30, had wrinkles at 35, dry skin at 40, joint stiffness at 45, high cholesterol by 50, heart disease at 55, memory loss at 57, and osteoporosis by 60! We don't have to live that life. To break the mold of aging, we must get healthy and live that way.

EXERCISE TIP

YOU MAKE ME FEEL LIKE DANCING. I'm telling you, there's nothing that makes you feel better than dancing. Think about how much fun you have when you go to a wedding. So today, we're not just going to put on music and dance. We're going to sign up for a dance class. Call up a studio and get a schedule. Maybe there's a dance that you've always wanted to learn, and you've been too embarrassed or too shy to take the class. Even if you have two left feet, there is nothing better than being able to dance.

153

I'm sure there's going to be some social function in your future when you're going to need to get up on the dance floor. So why not be a couple steps ahead of the game by signing up for a class now?

FOOD TIP

SOY TO THE RESCUE! The one thing you can always count on being in my refrigerator is a bowl of cooked soybeans. Get some frozen soybeans (edamame) from a grocery store. You can get them at a local health food store or in a Japanese market. Plunge them into salted boiling water for five minutes. You've got a great snack that will sustain you and combine with almost anything else that you eat. There are added benefits because we know how important soy is, especially for women.

DAY 14

BLUE

ORGANIZATIONAL TIP

JUNK THE JUNK MAIL. One of the worst piles of junk that accumulates in our house is the mail that stacks up on the kitchen counter. Unopened junk mail and solicitations can sit there for weeks before someone finally goes through them and throws them away. My new policy while writing this book has been to go through the mail as soon as it arrives, and throw away anything I don't need, deal immediately with anything that needs a response, or file away the rest. It's hard, but since adopting this discipline, I'm not forgetting to RSVP, and my counter is clutter-free. Even if you can't clean up your past piles right away, make it a point to start practicing this from today forward.

BEAUTY TIP

AVOID THE TAMMY FAYE LOOK. If you wear mascara, it's better to put it on in three layers. Let each layer dry thoroughly before you put on the next layer. There's nothing worse than being in a hurry and quickly putting on three layers without allowing drying time in between. Your eyelashes get squished together and full of black gunk. Then you have to comb through them. If you flake any mascara onto your base makeup, you'll have to start all over again, anyway. It's best to do it right, in stages, the first time.

SPA ON A BUDGET TIP

AND YOU THOUGHT IT WAS JUST A LAXATIVE! Whenever you have to wear makeup all day long, it's best to put a thin layer of castor oil on your face underneath your makeup to keep it fresh. I learned this tip from the wonderful makeup artist Anthony Lloyd, who did my face for *Noises Off* a few years ago. It was amazing. By the end of the day, my makeup didn't look cakey, and he kept saying that our secret was the castor oil. It was a very thin layer that felt very natural and didn't clog my pores at all. It holds the makeup beautifully, and it is so inexpensive.

TOTAL HEALTH FAKEOVER

BUT I'M NOT TIRED! Whenever I tell my boys it's time to go to bed, they always say, "But I'm not tired!" Children want to keep going and going. Sometimes as adults, we have to keep going, but it's not as if we want to. Well, today *want* to keep going, *want* to push yourself a little bit. Enjoy the fact that you're a grown-up, and you don't need a big nap in the middle of the day anymore. Fill up your day as much as you can and have the attitude that you don't want to miss anything. That's gusto. If you're dragging yourself through this, then it's not going to work. It's going to be so much worse for you. If you say, "Hey, you know what? I feel good!" then it's going to be a lot better.

Menu

DAY 14

Breakfast: 1½ cups of assorted fruits: pineapple, grapes, and/or strawberries. No melons and no bananas.

Lunch: Bel's Brown Rice and Veggies All in One

Snack: 2 handfuls of raw veggies and/or peppermint, red clover, chamomile, or burdock root tea

Dinner: Salad 101 (add chopped scallions) and Dressing 101, Whole Oven-Roasted Striped Bass with Olive Oil Infusion, Italian-Style Zucchini

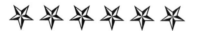

DAY 14

BLUE

Bel's Brown Rice and Veggies All in One — Lunch

SERVES 4

½ of a yellow or red bell pepper, diced

1 large carrot, diced

2 red plum tomatoes, seeded and diced

1 cup shredded cabbage

1 tablespoon olive oil

1 large clove garlic, pressed

1 cup brown rice

2½ cups water

Sauté all the vegetables in the oil. Add the garlic and brown rice. Sauté for another 3 to 5 minutes. Add the water, turn the heat to high, and boil all the water out. When all the water is gone, lower heat to *lowest setting*, place the lid on, and leave for 20 minutes. No peeking or stirring!

Salad 101 and Dressing 101 — Dinner

SERVES 2

- 1 tablespoon olive oil
- 1 teaspoon balsamic vinegar or white or red wine vinegar
- 1 teaspoon Dijon mustard
- 4 cups mixed greens
- 1 tomato, sliced
- 1 cucumber, sliced
- 2 scallions, chopped

DAY 14

BLUE

Combine the olive oil, vinegar, and mustard and mix well. Drizzle over the salad.

Whole Oven-Roasted Striped Bass with Olive Oil Infusion — Dinner

SERVES 4

- ½ cup extra virgin olive oil (superior quality)
- 1 pinch fennel seeds
- 1 pinch crushed red pepper flakes
- 2 sprigs thyme, minced
- 2 sage leaves, minced
- 1 sprig rosemary
- 4 whole striped bass (1¼ pounds each), gutted and scaled
- 2 fennel bulbs with tops, thinly sliced
- 4 cloves garlic, sliced
- Salt and pepper
- 4 vine-ripened tomatoes, sliced ¼ inch thick

Preheat the oven to 450 degrees. In a mixing bowl, combine the olive oil, fennel seeds, red pepper flakes, thyme, sage, and rosemary. Set aside. Stuff the belly of each fish with fennel and garlic. In a large baking pan, line the bottom with the rest of the sliced fennel and tops. Place each whole fish on the fennel and brush with one half of the olive oil/herb mixture. Season with salt and pepper. Place 4 to 5 tomato slices on top of each fish. Season the tomatoes with salt and pepper. Bake the whole fishes for 15 to 20 minutes.

Before serving, heat the remaining olive oil/herb mixture. On each plate, place a whole fish on a bed of fresh fennel. Drizzle mixture onto the fish.

Serge Falesitch
Executive Chef, L'Hermitage Hotel, Beverly Hills

DAY 14

BLUE

Italian-Style Zucchini—Dinner

SERVES 2

1 large or 2 small zucchini
½ to 1 teaspoon minced garlic
1 tablespoon olive oil
1 teaspoon dried basil
1 teaspoon dried oregano
½ teaspoon paprika
Freshly ground pepper

Use a food processor to cut the zucchini into thin ⅛-inch lengthwise strips. Combine the garlic and olive oil in a small bowl, then add the mixture to a large, non-stick skillet with the zucchini. Season with the herbs and paprika and sauté over medium-high heat, turning with tongs until the zucchini is bright green and al dente. Remove from the skillet and season to taste with pepper.

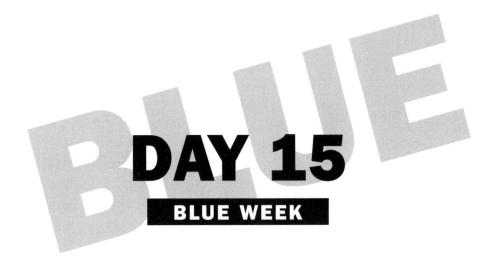

DAY 15

BLUE WEEK

MOTIVATIONAL TIP

THE 36-HOUR SOLUTION. Give any problem or drama 36 hours and watch it change. I can't tell you how many times I have seen this happen. You could almost set your watch by it. Whenever I get upset about something, 36 hours later, I have a completely different perspective. I don't know why 36 is the magic number, but it really is. It gives you time to digest it. It gives you time to stew in it. It gives you time to really come up with a "Plan B." It usually makes your life a lot easier. So don't rush to judgment. Don't rush to action. If something is a problem, give it a little time and watch it change. If it's not going to change in the universe, at least it may change in your mind so that you can change it in the universe for yourself.

EXERCISE TIP

HEAD FOR THE CENTER! Strengthen your center. Jay Grimes, my wonderful Pilates teacher, does this exercise once in a while. He tells me, "Whenever you feel like you've lost your center, lie on your back on the floor, get your knees up on a bed or a chair, and stay there for a while." You'll feel your back go against the floor and you'll become completely relaxed. And your center will be relocated to where it belongs. It's very important. It also strengthens your abdominal muscles, and it's a great position from which to do some crunches.

FOOD TIP

CRAVINGS, NOTHING MORE THAN CRAVINGS. We're almost halfway there, so what are we craving? Are we craving certain foods? Pay attention to what you may be craving at this point in the program. If you're not craving much, it's probably because you started from a good place to begin with. If you're having certain cravings , it might be that you're still cleaning out some sugar or dairy from your system. I've talked about food and mood before, but it's always a good subject to revisit. You're in a certain mood, you want a certain food. When you want to be comforted, you go back to the foods of your childhood. When you feel angry, you want to crunch on some peanuts. If you eat something too salty, you immediately want something sweet. You had something too sweet, you want something salty. Now that you're getting new foods, remember to keep writing in your food diary and make adjustments if you absolutely have to. Know that you're getting a nice balance of protein, starches, fats, and flavors on this program. Just be conscious of your cravings.

ORGANIZATIONAL TIP

SAVE TIME—BUY IN MULTIPLES. So much of our time is wasted looking for things, and it's usually looking for the *same* things. I was always looking for a pencil. I was always looking for paper. I was always looking for my sunglasses. I finally solved this by buying enough of them, and buying in bulk, which is always much cheaper. (I'm a real fan of Price Club and places like that.) If you buy the things you use a lot in multiples, you can then place them around your house, and you're not going to have to waste all your time looking for them. I can't tell you how much time it has saved me, not only time searching but also time being aggravated.

BEAUTY TIP

REMOVE EXCESS BUILDUP ON YOUR HAIR. Fill a liter-sized water bottle ⅔ full of white vinegar and ⅓ full of water. Use it after shampooing and before applying your conditioner to remove excess buildup on your hair. Do this once a month and it will keep you from having to buy an expensive detoxifying shampoo or from having to rotate your shampoos. It's especially good to do right *before* you're going to color your hair. Just make sure you use a nice, strong conditioner afterwards.

SPA ON A BUDGET

HE SAID, SHE SAID. We always have all these products in our bathroom, and guys could use them, too, but they never know what to use them for. We can use baby powder for chafing (it isn't just for babies, you know), or it can also be used to freshen up unwashed sheets for those "unexpected" sleepovers! He can use your hair conditioner as shaving cream, hair thickener to buff his shoes, or mascara to cover up some unwanted gray hair (on his moustache or eyebrows). Petroleum jelly can even work as an emergency hair gel.

DAY 15

BLUE

TOTAL HEALTH FAKEOVER

SHOP, BUT DON'T DROP ANY MONEY! Go shopping, but don't spend any money. Don't even bring your credit cards with you. Check out what's out there. See what the current fashions are. See what they're showing on mannequins. Try on some new styles and get a sense of where you are *right now* with your body and what's current. Next week we're going to spend a lot of time in our closets. Who knows? Maybe what's in the stores is already in there.

Menu

DAY 15

On Rising: 6 ounces of fruit juice or 1 piece of seasonal fruit

Breakfast: (2 hours after rising) Mary Ann's Corn Muffins

Lunch: Cold Salmon Salad

Snack: 2 handfuls of raw veggies and/or one of the usual teas

Dinner: Shrimp and Veggie Stir-fry

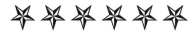

DAY 15

BLUE

Mary Ann's Corn Muffins — Breakfast

SERVES 8

½ cup corn oil
2 egg whites
½ cup maple syrup
1½ cups water
2 cups cornmeal
2 cups whole wheat pastry flour
4 teaspoons baking powder
Poppy seeds, optional

DAY 15

BLUE Preheat the oven to 375 degrees. Mix the liquid ingredients. Sift the dry ingredients separately. Combine the wet and dry ingredients. You should be able to pour the batter. Spoon into muffin cups or an oiled muffin pan. Bake 20 minutes. The tops of the muffins should crack slightly.

Cold Salmon Salad — Lunch

SERVES 4

1 pound salmon fillet
2 tablespoons stone-ground mustard
1 tablespoon chopped fresh basil or ¾ teaspoon dried basil

Preheat the broiler. Set oven rack 4 to 5 inches from the element. Rinse the fish, pat it dry, and lay it skin-side down on a baking sheet. Mix the mustard and basil. Brush the mixture over the salmon. Broil the salmon until it's opaque in the center, about 5 to 6 minutes for a ½-inch-thick fillet or 10 to 12 minutes for a 1-inch fillet. Serve hot or cold over Salad 101 with Dressing 101 (see page 158).

Shrimp and Veggie Stir-fry — Dinner

SERVES 4

1 tablespoon toasted sesame oil

½ cabbage, chopped

1 large carrot, julienned

1 medium yellow onion, cut in chunks

½ yellow pepper, thinly sliced lengthwise

½ red pepper, thinly sliced lengthwise

1 teaspoon minced fresh ginger

1 medium clove garlic, minced

2 teaspoons tamari

1 teaspoon toasted sesame seeds

½ pound shrimp, deveined

DAY 15

BLUE

In a very hot wok or large pan, put the oil and all the vegetables and seasonings all at once and stir-fry, constantly stirring, over high heat for 4 to 5 minutes. Take out the vegetables with a slotted spoon and set aside. Put the shrimp in the remaining juices and stir-fry till cooked. Add the vegetables and toss together. Serve hot. Remember, we're food combining, so no rice! Leave ½ cup of the stir-fry for breakfast tomorrow.

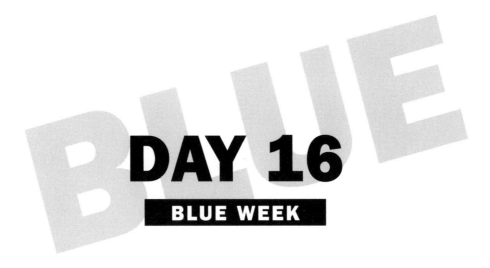

DAY 16
BLUE WEEK

MOTIVATIONAL TIP

WHENEVER YOU HAVE A MEETING, AN INTERVIEW, OR A DOCTOR'S APPOINTMENT, KNOW WHAT YOU WANT TO ACCOMPLISH. How many times have you left an important meeting with someone only to realize that you didn't achieve what you had originally set out to accomplish? It's best to know your purpose. Know your agenda. Write it down if you have to, or write down the questions you want answered and make sure you get your answers. We often get distracted by the other person's agenda or personality and fail to make our point. Try not to let that happen. Prepare yourself so that you get the most out of every encounter.

EXERCISE TIP

EXERCISE YOUR MEMORY. One of the most important things we can exercise is our memory. I play memory games with my kids all the time. I'm always exercising my mind. For example, before I go shopping, I imagine myself in the grocery store, and I try to make my grocery list according to the aisles. The next time you go shopping, play that memory game. Write out your grocery list according to the aisles, and then see how close you come.

FOOD TIP

THESE ARE A FEW OF MY FAVORITE CUISINES. People tend to think of health food as a separate cuisine. What you *should* do is take healthy food and turn it into your favorite cuisine by adding the following herbs and spices.

Mexican
Fresh cilantro, fresh green onion, fresh bell pepper, fresh limes, cumin, jalapeño pepper flakes, Mexican oregano

Italian
Tarragon, basil, garlic, pine nuts, extra virgin olive oil, fennel, thyme, Italian parsley, rosemary, balsamic vinegar, sun-dried tomatoes

Chinese
Five spice, soy sauce, any Chinese rice wine vinegar, fresh ginger

Indian
Curry, cayenne, cardamom, garlic masala, turmeric, cinnamon, tahini

Japanese
Mirin, rice vinegar, soy sauce (different variations), miso, ginger, sesame oil, sesame seeds, nori

ORGANIZATIONAL TIP

HAMPER DAY TIP #1. Years ago, when I was dating John Travolta, one of the things we both had in common was that we came from big families. We always made this joke about how hanging out at our families' houses was like hanging out in a big hamper. "Hamper" consequently became known as anything that was a little off. For example, I'd say, "This blouse is really hamper," because it would be an expensive blouse but it would have a little grease stain on it, so I'd put a pin over the spot. I'd say "Oh my gosh, these sunglasses are so hamper." The screw had come off, and instead of replacing the screw there was a little gold safety pin holding it together. Or in the old days when I wore a school uniform, I'd put safety pins or sometimes even staples to fix a tear instead of having it sewn. You get the idea. Hamper is anything that's a little off or hasn't been properly fixed. Rather than taking the time to fix it, you end up patching it together somehow. Today, we're going to try to be less hamper. Anything about us that's hamper we're going to try to fix. This is going to be hamper day. Better yet, it's non-hamper day.

BEAUTY TIP

DAY 16

BLUE

TWEEZE, PLEASE—HAMPER DAY TIP #2. De-hamper that body of yours. Get rid of all those wandering hairs you find from your eyebrows to your toes. You know, the ones that don't belong to any particular place or thing. Those who, what, when, where, how hairs—*Who* are you? *What* are you doing here? *When* did you get here? *Where* did you come from? *How* can I get rid of you? Say good-bye to those straggly strangers—pluck 'em, wax 'em, shave 'em, dump 'em.

SPA ON A BUDGET.

FADE TO BLACK—HAMPER DAY TIP #3. Nothing will make your black clothes look more hamper than a dull fade to gray. To avoid this, add a cup of white vinegar to the rinse cycle of the wash to keep your dark color clothing rich and dark. We do this in my house all the time, and it's amazing.

TOTAL HEALTH FAKEOVER

HAMPER DAY TIP #4. Not only are we going to clean up the little things we use personally every day, but we're going to start paying attention to everything else. Make a mental checklist of all the things that you use in your life. If you go to pick up the phone, and the cord is so bad you have to hold it a certain way to get it to work, think about getting a new cord! A touch of the hamper is never bad. It's actually desirable because it makes you very real. But if everything in your life is hamper, you might want to look into changing it.

Menu

DAY 16

On Rising: 6 ounces of fruit juice or 1 piece of seasonal fruit

Breakfast: (2 hours after fruit) Egg White Stir-fry

Lunch: Tangy Fusilli Pasta Salad

Snack: 2 handfuls of raw veggies and/or one of the usual teas

Dinner: Seaweed Sesame Salad, Wolfgang Puck's Striped Bass in Ginger Vinaigrette with side of steamed broccoli

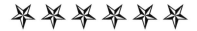

DAY 16

BLUE

Egg White Stir-fry—Breakfast

SERVES 1

Olive oil spray
3 egg whites
½ cup leftover stir-fry from dinner, Day 15

Coat the pan with olive oil spray. Scramble the egg whites with the leftover stir-fry. Cook in pan over medium heat.

DAY 16

BLUE

Tangy Fusilli Pasta Salad—Lunch

SERVES 4

1 pound fusilli pasta
1 cup favorite all-natural, non-dairy balsamic vinaigrette
2 large cloves garlic, minced
¼ cup chopped fresh basil
1 zucchini, sliced into half moons
1 medium carrot, diced
4 scallions, thinly sliced
½ cup cauliflower, small florets
½ cup broccoli, small florets
¼ cup thinly sliced mushrooms
1 can artichoke hearts in water, drained and roughly chopped
½ cup sun-dried tomatoes, drained and sliced (optional as garnish)

In a large covered stockpot, bring 4 quarts of water to a boil. Add the pasta and cook for 12 to 15 minutes or until *al dente*. Pour into a strainer and run under cold water until cool. Drain thoroughly. In a large bowl, combine the pasta with the balsamic vinaigrette and toss until pasta is evenly coated.

Add the remaining ingredients, except for the optional sun-dried tomatoes, and mix well. Cover and let sit, refrigerated, for at least 2 hours, or preferably overnight. Before serving, garnish with the sun-dried tomatoes, if desired.

Seaweed Sesame Salad–Dinner

SERVES 6

2 cups dry arame (a type of seaweed)
4 cloves garlic, minced
1 tablespoon minced ginger
2 carrots, sliced into matchstick pieces
2 teaspoons toasted sesame oil
¼ cup rice vinegar
2 tablespoons honey
2 tablespoons tamari
4 scallions, shredded
2 tablespoons sesame seeds
½ cup daikon, sliced into matchstick pieces
½ cup red bell pepper, sliced into matchstick pieces
Boston or romaine lettuce

DAY 16

BLUE

Soak the arame in hot water for 15 minutes. Drain and place in a saucepan with the garlic, ginger, carrots, and enough water to cover. Bring to a boil and cook until the arame and carrots are just tender. Drain immediately and place in a mixing bowl.

Combine the oil, vinegar, honey, tamari, and scallions. Pour over the arame and mix well. Stir in the sesame seeds, daikon, and bell pepper and toss. Serve the salad on a bed of Boston or romaine lettuce.

Wolfgang Puck's Striped Bass in Ginger Vinaigrette — Dinner

SERVES 4

One of my all-time favorite chefs was nice enough to give me this healthy, delicious recipe. You could also use red snapper in this recipe.

DAY 16

BLUE

1 1-inch piece ginger, peeled and minced

2 large shallots, minced

¼ cup rice wine vinegar

⅓ cup extra virgin olive oil

Juice of 2 limes

2 tablespoons soy sauce

2 tablespoons toasted sesame oil

Salt

Freshly ground white pepper

4 striped bass fillets, 6 ounces each

1 bunch cilantro or Italian parsley, roughly chopped, plus a few whole leaves for garnish

¼ cup toasted sesame seeds for garnish

Combine the ginger, shallots, vinegar, olive oil, lime juice, and soy sauce in a small bowl. Whisking vigorously, add the sesame oil and salt and pepper to taste. Season the striped bass on both sides with salt and pepper. Grill it over high heat until done or sauté it in a little soy margarine or oil. Striped bass fillets that are ½ inch thick take only 1 to 2 minutes on each side. Just before serving, mix the cilantro or parsley into the vinaigrette. (This prevents the herbs from turning dark.)

For presentation, make a pool of the vinaigrette on the dinner plates at room temperature. Top with the grilled fish. Garnish with the toasted sesame seeds and a few cilantro or parsley leaves. Serve with steamed broccoli.

Wolfgang Puck
Spago, Beverly Hills

DAY 16

BLUE

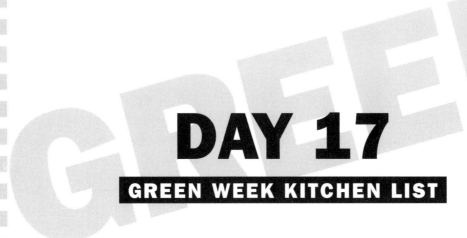

DAY 17

GREEN WEEK KITCHEN LIST

Everything you will need for Green Week's menus

Check your kitchen for what you already have. Check recipes for amounts.

Vegetables

Asparagus
Avocado
Beefsteak or extra large
  tomatoes
Bell peppers: red, yellow,
  green
Bok choy
Broccoli
Carrots
Cauliflower
Celery
Corn kernels, frozen
Corn on the cob
Cucumber
Garlic, fresh
Green beans

Italian plum tomatoes,
  canned
Jalapeños
Kabocha squash
Mushrooms
Onions: red, yellow, white
Peas, frozen
Plum tomatoes
Romaine lettuce
Scallions
Serrano chilies
Shallots
Shiitake mushrooms
Spinach
Tomatoes
Water chestnuts
Watercress

Yellow plum tomatoes
Yellow wax beans
Zucchini

Grains, Breads, Pasta

Arborio rice
Bread crumbs
Brown rice
Cornmeal
Flourless whole grain bread
Linguine
Oatmeal
Pasta: penne, shells,
  spaghetti, or linguine
Ready-to-cook pizza crust

174

Protein
Ahi tuna (highest grade)
Chilean sea bass
Eggs
Salmon fillet
Sea bass
Tuna (highest grade)

Legumes
Edamame (soybeans)
Garbanzo beans,
    canned
Great Northern beans,
    canned
Lentils
White beans, dry

Herbs & Spices
Baking powder
Basil, dried
Basil, fresh
Bay leaf
Black pepper
Chives
Cilantro, fresh
Cinnamon
Crushed red pepper flakes
Fennel seeds
Garlic
Ginger

Gomasio (a Japanese
    condiment)
Mint, fresh
No-salt Italian herb
    seasoning blend
Oregano, dried
Oregano, fresh
Parsley, fresh
Poppy seeds
Powdered saffron
Rosemary, fresh
Sea salt
Sesame seeds
Thyme, dried
Thyme, fresh
Vanilla extract
White pepper

Fruits & Juices
Juices of choice
Lemon
Lime or lime juice
Seasonal fruit

Miscellaneous
Artichoke hearts, canned
Barley malt
Black olives
Canola oil
Corn oil

Curry sauce
Dijon mustard
Extra virgin olive oil
Fish stock or clam juice
Honey
Horseradish
Maple syrup
Mirin
Natural Italian dressing
Natural pizza sauce
Nayonaise
No oil corn chips
Nori (Seaweed)
Parchment paper
Peanut oil
Rice Dream
Rice vinegar
Salsa
Sesame oil
Soy cheese
Soy Parmesan cheese
Soy sauce
Sun-dried tomatoes
Tamari
Tofu, firm or extra firm
Tofu, soft
Vegetable broth
Vegetable spray
Wasabi powder
Water chestnuts

DAY 17

GREEN

MOTIVATIONAL TIP

THE KEY TO YOUR LIFE IS HOW WELL YOU DEAL WITH "PLAN B." You can aim for "Plan A." You can plan on "Plan A." But "Plan B" is what actually happens to you. It's your resilience in being able to roll with the punches and move on to "Plan B" that really makes your life. If something doesn't work out, don't automatically think that something bad has happened. Think of it as a new opportunity. Think of it as "Plan B." You never know why things happen the way they happen, but that's life. That's how it unfolds. When it happens that way, don't feel like you have to be dragged kicking and screaming into "Plan B," because sometimes "Plan B" is so much better. This is definitely the number one theory I live by.

EXERCISE TIP

EXERCISE FORGIVENESS. Sometimes you have to forgive yourself or someone else. The lack of forgiveness toward someone or something in your environment will often hold you back. It's important to forgive and move on. It's part of Plan B. The way this could apply to this program is the following: If you've been less than perfect, don't beat yourself up for it. Forgive yourself, resolve to do better, and move on.

DAY 17

GREEN

FOOD TIP

WATERMAN. Spend the entire day making water your only beverage. Notice how much better you digest your food. We couldn't do this all the time because that would be pretty boring, but try it at least for today. Don't gulp it with your meals but remember to drink a lot of water between meals. When I was on David Letterman's show the night before New Year's Eve '97, he and I talked about how our New Year's resolution was to drink only water during the day. He had done it for a couple of days already and noticed that it really worked for him. It's funny, the days that I do it I don't even think about any other beverage, and I always have an easier time digesting my food.

ORGANIZATIONAL TIP

AMNESTY DAY. When I was a kid in Chicago, January 2nd was the day every year that the library allowed you to take all of your books back, and you weren't charged for it. So on January 1st we would gather up the books that we hadn't returned to take them back the next day. Today is the day that you should do the same kind of thing. Walk around your house, and if there's anything that you're supposed to return to a neighbor, give it back to them. We all have those things buried in our house that we have borrowed. Somewhere a generous friend is missing them.

BEAUTY TIP

STEAM HEAT. One of the most important things we can do is to keep ourselves moist, both inside and out. I grew up in Chicago, and I can't tell you how different my skin is now from when I was living with radiators. When I discovered a humidifier, it made all the difference in my hair, my skin, and around my eyes. A lot of people don't realize that when you have fake heat at home, like a radiator, or if you live in a dry climate, it's constantly sucking moisture from your system. Keep a lot of moisture in the air by buying a humidifier. Having lots of plants around your house is also a good idea.

SPA ON A BUDGET

TAKE A SLENDERIZING BATH WITH BAKING SODA. Fill your tub half full with warm water, add 1 cup of baking soda, fill the tub the rest of the way. Soak for 20 minutes. Add your favorite fragrance. Do this 10 consecutive days. It enhances weight loss, reduces toxins, and makes your skin feel baby smooth. This is something my sister-in-law Lynnette tried while we were working on this book, and she couldn't believe the difference in her body. Now, she's a tub soaker and loves doing this every day.

TOTAL HEALTH FAKEOVER

DON'T THROW A PITY PARTY. DO SOMETHING NICE FOR SOMEONE ELSE. This is something I have tried to live by my entire life. Whenever I feel sorry for myself, I always try to do something constructive with the feeling. I try to turn it around and say, "I know I'm feeling bad, but if I do something to make somebody else feel good, I could probably make myself feel better as well." It could be any number of things. You can look around and find something in your environment that somebody else would really like. If you don't have anyone in your immediate circle, there are so many other people out there, strangers who could use your help, even if it's on a volunteer basis: older people, sick people, or people in a shelter.

Menu

DAY 17

On Rising: 6 ounces fruit juice or 1 piece of seasonal fruit

Breakfast: (2 hours after fruit) Joey's French Toast

Lunch: White Bean Soup

Dinner: Stir-fry Spaghetti

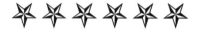

DAY 17

GREEN

Joey's French Toast — Breakfast

SERVES 1

1 egg white with splash of rice milk
Dash vanilla extract
Dash cinnamon
1 slice flourless, whole-grain bread
½ teaspoon maple syrup

Combine the egg white, rice milk, vanilla, and cinnamon in a bowl. Whisk well. Dip the bread thoroughly into the liquid, coating well, and cook on a nonstick griddle or in a pan lightly greased with soy margarine. You can now drizzle on the maple syrup.

DAY 17

GREEN

White Bean Soup — Lunch

SERVES 4 TO 6

4 cups dry white beans soaked overnight in 6 cups of water
½ cup minced carrots
½ cup minced onions
½ cup minced celery
¼ teaspoon minced garlic
¼ cup light olive oil
1 bay leaf
8 cups water
1 teaspoon sea salt
½ teaspoon black pepper
½ teaspoon minced thyme

DAY 17

GREEN

Strain the soaked beans in a colander. Then, in a large pot, sauté the carrots, onions, celery, and garlic in the olive oil over medium heat. After the vegetables are lightly cooked, add the beans and bay leaf and water and bring to a boil. Reduce to a simmer and cook for 1 hour, or until the beans are cooked all the way through. Add the salt, pepper, and thyme.

Lance Correlez
Taix Restaurant, Los Angeles

Stir-fry Spaghetti — Dinner

SERVES 6

1 pound spaghetti or linguine

2 teaspoons extra virgin olive oil

2 cups broccoli, small florets

2 red bell peppers, julienned

1 pound firm tofu, well-drained and diced into 1-inch cubes

3 large mushrooms, thinly sliced

1 cup chopped fresh basil

1 cup thinly sliced black olives

3 large cloves garlic, minced

1 cup bottled natural Italian salad dressing

½ teaspoon freshly ground black pepper

2 teaspoons no-salt Italian herbal seasoning blend

⅓ cup grated soy Parmesan, optional

DAY 17

GREEN

In a large, covered stockpot, bring 4 quarts of water to a boil. Add the pasta and cook for 12 to 15 minutes or until *al dente*. Pour into a strainer and reserve. Heat a wok or large sauté pan over high heat until almost smoking. Add the olive oil and stir-fry the broccoli for 2 to 3 minutes, stirring constantly. Add the red bell peppers and stir-fry 1 minute longer. Add the tofu, mushrooms, basil, olives, and garlic and stir-fry for 1 minute. Stir in the salad dressing, pepper, and Italian herb blend. Add the reserved pasta and toss until the ingredients are evenly incorporated and the pasta is heated through. Serve immediately with soy Parmesan on top, if desired.

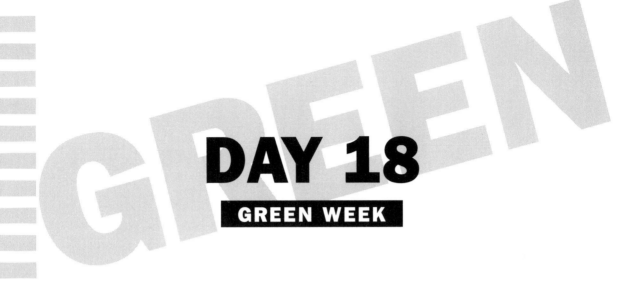

DAY 18

GREEN WEEK

MOTIVATIONAL TIP

ACCENTUATE THE POSITIVE. Okay, it's week three. We're getting in better and better shape. Remember when I talked to you about your assets and liabilities—the good will get great and the bad will get better? What I want you to do today is focus on a body part that you love, whether it's your legs, your arms, or your waist. "Celebrate" that body part. Dress for it and show it off. It's usually the first part of you that gets into shape. It's important to accentuate the positive and to work it.

EXERCISE TIP

SET YOUR WALK TO MUSIC. I love to walk. I also love to listen to music while I'm moving. Some of the tapes that I've used over the years include classics like Prince's "1999" and "Purple Rain" and Bryan Ferry's "Boy and Girls." Paul Simon's "Graceland" is a great walking album. Anything by the Pet Shop Boys or the Gypsy Kings is good for walking. I love old disco, which has become popular again. Most recently Sheryl Crow, Madonna, and Jamiroquai keep me moving. Sometimes I go for instrumental albums by Robert Miles. If you want to, listen to books on tape as well. (Especially my books!)

FOOD TIP

THE SEVEN ESSENTIALS TO BEING GOURMET READY. I asked one of my favorite cooks what she always has in her refrigerator. She said you could turn any dish into a gourmet meal if, like a Girl Scout, you were always prepared with seven foods. Those seven are green onions, plum tomatoes, cilantro, dill, lime, grated carrots, and beets. It's best if they're fresh. These foods are so life-giving that you don't even need to cook them. There's great energy in each one of them, and the variety of dishes you can prepare is limitless.

ORGANIZATIONAL TIP

EVERYTHING IN ITS PLACE. The best way to organize is to make sure that everything has a place (and I don't mean the back of a chair or the top of a counter). There are always those places where things tend to accumulate. Avoid this by temporarily getting rid of that spot: i.e., removing that chair from its usual location or temporarily covering the area with something else. (Who knows, maybe under that pile of clothes you'll find a treadmill or a StairMaster!) I have a director's chair in my bathroom where things tend to pile up. When I remove the chair, it forces me to put everything away. Once I know I'm in the groove of putting things back, I can bring that chair back.

DAY 18

GREEN

BEAUTY TIP

MAKE FRIENDS WITH "YOUR FRIEND." One of the most important things we can learn about the natural flow of life is learning how to embrace our menstrual cycle. It happens to us every month. The next time you feel it coming on, understand that it's part of the ebb and flow of your life cycle. It's not something to be feared or irritated over because it's just a normal part of a woman's life. You're eating better, so it's probably not going to affect you quite as much. I used to have terrible PMS. After years of being aggravated by it, I finally found a cure that worked for me. I realized that it was best to have centered foods the five days before, and not to give in to those extreme salt and sugar cravings. Don't even give in once. Don't have candy. Don't have salty potato chips. That'll just start the whole cycle of extreme cravings. Don't drink any alcohol, either. Try to get plenty of rest and exercise. It's a good way to live anyway.

SPA ON A BUDGET

EVERYTHING OLD IS NEW AGAIN. Nothing can make you look more put together than shoes or a handbag that looks new. And a lot of times we have those things. We just don't realize it. Take your old leather goods to a shoe repair, and they will do everything. They'll fix straps, handles, shoes, heels, and will dye your things. Freshening up a great pair of shoes that have already been broken in will certainly make it easier on your feet and your back. Also, if you've bought a bag in a wild color that you don't wear that often, have it dyed basic black or brown. You'll get a lot more use out of it.

DAY 18

GREEN

TOTAL HEALTH FAKEOVER

DAMAGE CONTROL DAY. This is where we try to put fires out before they even happen. Try to anticipate anything that's about to go haywire. You're probably feeling better, have more control, and are better organized in your life now, so you can have your antenna focused outward. Have your radar set higher than you normally would for potential danger. Anticipate and fix the problem before it all falls apart. Instead of giving in to the toxicity of the relationships either at home or at work, rise above it and be the negotiator. A lot of times in show business, people are working close together and tempers often flare at the slightest provocation. It's so important to stay calm and centered during those volatile times.

Menu

DAY 18

On Rising: 6 ounces of fruit juice or 1 piece of seasonal fruit

Breakfast: Nicky's Favorite Oatmeal

Lunch: Seared Rare Ahi Tuna with a Three-Bean and Tomato Salad

Dinner: Vegetable Paella

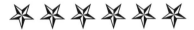

DAY 18

GREEN

Nicky's Favorite Oatmeal — Breakfast

SERVES 1

½ cup oatmeal (quick)
¾ cup boiling water
½ teaspoon maple syrup

Put the oatmeal in a bowl, add the boiling water, and drizzle with maple syrup.

Seared Rare Ahi Tuna with a Three-Bean and Tomato Salad—Lunch

SERVES 4

For the marinade

2 tablespoons rice vinegar
2 tablespoons soy sauce
½ teaspoon toasted sesame seeds
1 shallot, finely sliced
1 tablespoon chopped cilantro

For the Salad

¼ cup sliced red plum tomatoes
¼ cup sliced yellow plum tomatoes
1 cup yellow wax beans, stemmed and blanched
1 cup green beans, stemmed and blanched
¼ cup edamame (soybeans), shelled and blanched
Vegetable spray
4 very fresh sushi-grade Ahi tuna fillets, 5 ounces each
1 bunch watercress, cleaned and stemmed, for garnish

DAY 18

GREEN

Preheat the oven to 400 degrees. In a medium bowl, mix the marinade ingredients and let sit for at least 4 minutes. Add the tomatoes and beans to the marinade and let sit, covered in plastic wrap, for at least 30 minutes.

In a very hot sauté pan held away from the flame, spray enough vegetable spray to coat the pan. Return to the heat and sear the tuna over high heat until golden brown, about 2 minutes on each side. Place the pan in the preheated oven for about 3 minutes to finish the cooking.

To serve, divide the watercress among the centers of 4 plates. Divide the three-bean and tomato salad on top of the watercress bed. Slice the tuna in half on the bias and place on top of the salad. Serve immediately.

Vegetable Paella — Dinner

SERVES 4

⅓ **cup water**
1 **onion, chopped**
1½ **teaspoons minced fresh garlic**
4 **cups vegetable broth**
½ **teaspoon white pepper**
¼ **teaspoon powdered saffron**
1 **cup arborio rice**
2 **cups cut green beans**
2 **zucchini, cut in half lengthwise, then sliced**
1 **red bell pepper, cut into strips**
1 **or 2 ears corn, cut into 1-inch pieces**
1 **tablespoon minced fresh basil**
1 **tablespoon minced fresh parsley**
¼ **teaspoon grated lemon zest**
1 **15-ounce can garbanzo beans, drained and rinsed**
1 **14-ounce can artichoke hearts, drained and rinsed**

DAY 18

GREEN

Place the water, onion, and garlic in a large saucepan. Cook, stirring frequently, for 3 minutes. Add the broth, pepper, and saffron. Bring to a boil and stir in the rice and green beans. Reduce the heat, cover, and cook over low heat for 8 minutes. Add the zucchini, bell pepper, corn, basil, parsley, and lemon zest. Mix well. Cover and cook for an additional 8 minutes. Add the garbanzo beans and artichoke hearts. Cook, stirring occasionally, for about 5 minutes. Serve hot.

DAY 19

GREEN WEEK

MOTIVATIONAL TIP

PASSION EQUALS ENERGY. The more I want to get something done, the less I call it work. The more focused you are on a task at hand, the more energy you'll put toward it and the more you'll keep your eye on the ball. Many people in the middle of a job cannot move forward because they're always looking around and trying to find excuses to get out of what they have to do. This makes it a real drudgery. If you can find the joy in something, you're not only going to put a lot more energy into it, you're going to get it done a lot faster.

EXERCISE TIP

LEARN WHERE YOU CAN FIRM. Put aside some time today to research all your exercise possibilities. Call health clubs, dancing schools, college recreation departments, community centers, and so on. Tell them to send you schedules, location maps, prices, and anything else you will need to explore new exercise outlets.

FOOD TIP

SPICE UP YOUR LIFE. Like the seven essentials for being gourmet ready, the following spices will keep your kitchen prepared for any occasion. Stock the following dry herbs and spices in your cabinet:

Dill

Lemon pepper

Basil

Garlic powder

Cilantro

Oregano

Paprika

Italian spices

I also love some of the seasonings that don't have MSG, available at health food stores. Spike, VegeSal, and Gomasio are just a few examples.

ORGANIZATIONAL TIP

HANGING TOGETHER. I've been waiting for this tip! This is the whole reason I wanted to do a book. I wanted to get in people's closets and help them organize it. This is something I could do professionally. After being an actress and an author, I'm really a "closet" organizer. (I don't mean a secret organizer, because by now you know I'm loud and proud to be organized!) Okay, look at your closet. Is there any available space? Are things so piled up that you can't find them anyway? The most important thing to do is make sure that everything has a place in your closet. This sometimes means getting wire baskets, a shoe rack, or hanging things on the back of the door. Most people don't have big closets, so you have to use every available space. No matter what kind of apartment I was in, my closet was always organized. Look around and see if things can be better organized in terms of hanging the clothes that are alike together. (Hang pants together, hang blouses together, and so on) Most people just shove their clothes in the closet, but that makes them so much harder to find. I'm looking to save you time. If you can get it organized to begin with, you're going to save a lot more time further down the road. You're not going to be scrambling around every morning looking for things.

BEAUTY TIP

PUT YOUR BODY TO BED. I probably exhausted you today with organizing your closet or just *thinking* about your closet. So here's a little sleep trick I figured out when I was six years old. As I've told you several times, I was never much of a sleeper. One thing that always helps me sleep is thinking about every part of my body and relaxing it, starting with the toes. It's like your toes become completely dead weight, then your feet, then your ankles. Move on up your body and stay completely still, as though you're putting every part of your body to sleep. I rarely make it past my hips. I never use my bed for anything except—well, two things, I guess. I don't read in bed because I'll associate my bed with another activity besides the two important ones. I make jokes all the time about having trouble falling asleep. So I'll say to my husband, "Tell me what you did today, honey." As he starts talking, it'll sort of lull me into sleep. (Not that his stories are boring . . . wink, wink.)

SPA ON A BUDGET TIP

DAY 19

GREEN

MASSAGE BUDDIES. Turn your partner into a massage buddy. Make appointments with each other. There are so many oils you can use, even a little bit of almond or peanut oil from your kitchen. Or you can buy a massage oil. They're not very expensive, and they will really make a difference in the quality of the massage you give and get. Make sure there's a pillow under your knees if you're lying flat on your back. Decide which part you like to start with first. When I get a massage, I know that I carry the most tension in my feet. If my feet are worked on first, I know that everything else will relax. Maybe you've never had a massage before, and it's something that feels too indulgent for you. Know that massage can be very therapeutic. It's not just a beauty treatment. Our muscles store lactic acid and by massaging them, it will make you feel better and less toxic. You will feel relaxed and more balanced as a result. A massage should really become part of your regular health routine.

TOTAL HEALTH FAKEOVER

THE BEST YOU FOR YOU. You don't have to dress for anybody else today. Today is the day that you're going to put on your clothes and make a great presentation just for yourself. Sometimes the best person to pull it all together for is *you*. If I'm working hard and haven't taken enough time for myself, sometimes cleaning up, putting on a little makeup even when I don't have to, fixing my hair, and wearing something besides sweats makes me feel like a whole new person. If you have to go to two places today, instead of just layering on makeup or throwing on dirty clothes, clean yourself up. Make a presentation. Be the best you for you.

Menu

DAY 19

On Rising: 6 ounces of fruit juice or 1 piece of seasonal fruit

Breakfast: (2 hours after fruit) Scrambled egg white with soy cheese

Lunch: Bel's Pasta Salad

Dinner: Spicy Chickpea Salad, Cilantro-Lime Sea Bass

DAY 19

GREEN

Scrambled Egg Whites with Soy Cheese — Breakfast

SERVES 1

3 egg whites
1 slice soy cheese, any flavor
1 slice whole grain toast with 1 pat soy margarine

Coat the pan with olive oil spray. Scramble the egg whites over medium heat, adding the soy cheese. Serve with toast and margarine.

Bel's Pasta Salad — Lunch

SERVES 4

DAY 19

GREEN

4 cups penne pasta, cooked
2 fresh zucchinis, grated
1 carrot, grated
1 cup frozen peas, thawed
½ medium red onion, finely sliced
1 cucumber, diced, optional

Dressing

1½ tablespoons canola oil
1 teaspoon rice vinegar

¼ teaspoon Dijon mustard
¼ teaspoon fresh minced garlic

In a large bowl, toss all ingredients.

Spicy Chickpea Salad — Dinner

SERVES 6

3 cups cooked chickpeas (garbanzo beans)
1 cucumber, peeled, seeded, and diced
¼ cup chopped fresh mint or cilantro
¾ cup reserved bean cooking liquid
1 small red onion, diced
1 serrano or jalapeño pepper, minced
3 tablespoons lime juice
4 teaspoons honey
2 teaspoons minced ginger root
2 teaspoons minced garlic
1 teaspoon crushed fennel seeds
¼ teaspoon salt

Combine the chickpeas, cucumber, and mint or cilantro in a large mixing bowl and set aside. In a small saucepan, combine the remaining ingredients. Bring to a boil, reduce the heat, and cook 15 minutes or until half the liquid remains. Immediately pour the sauce over the chickpeas. Toss to coat. Cover and refrigerate for at least 2 hours, stirring occasionally.

DAY 19

GREEN

Cilantro-Lime Sea Bass — Dinner

SERVES 1

6 to 8 ounces Chilean sea bass
1 tablespoon lime juice
1 tablespoon cilantro
1 teaspoon minced shallots
¼ teaspoon olive oil
Salt and pepper to taste

Preheat the oven to 375 degrees. Tear off parchment paper to make a square, then fold in half to make a triangle. Open the paper and place the fish inside at the fold. In a small bowl, mix the lime juice, cilantro, shallots, and olive oil together and pour over the fish. Season with salt and pepper to taste. Seal the paper tightly all the way around. Cook for 15 to 20 minutes, depending on thickness.

DAY 19

GREEN

DAY 20

GREEN WEEK

MOTIVATIONAL TIP

RAISE THE BAR. I have this theory that you should always aim high in life because most of the time you're really only going to get about 65 percent of what you aim for. If your aim is low, then 65 percent of that is not very much. If you aim really high, 65 percent of that will be like everyone else's 100 percent. So here we are, at around 65 percent of the way there. How's your aim?

EXERCISE TIP

MUST-SEE-TV WORKOUT. I don't know what day you started this program. But if today is Thursday, Monday, or Sunday, if you're watching television this evening, do some form of exercise during the commercials. Find little pockets of time during your TV watching, and do some buttocks tucks, leg lifts, or whatever. Do something physical during commercials, just for the heck of it. You'll have probably ten minutes during an hour's worth of television, and maybe you can even break a sweat.

FOOD TIP

AVOID STARVATION. Anytime on this program or in the future that you find yourself having to eat late at night, figure out what you should eat in the meantime. This will keep you from being so ravenous that you'll pig out when you finally get to your dinner. I recommend deciding what kind of meal you're going to be having later that night, whether it's a starch or a protein meal. It's best to have a little bit of that kind of food earlier so when you're eating dinner two hours later, you won't be mis-combining. Make sure you always have something in your car in case you're going to be driving long distances or you're not going to get home in time to eat. You should also have some bottled water in your car. I know with my children I have healthy snacks around so if they get hungry, there's always a little something for them to munch on. I know for myself I need that as well. Make sure you don't get so hungry on this diet that you eat the wrong foods.

ORGANIZATIONAL TIP

AN EXTRA PAIR PER SHELF! Organize your shoes in your closet by alternating each shoe's direction. Friends keep teasing me about this tip, but it really helps. Face each shoe in opposite directions, and you will gain enough space for an extra pair of shoes. This is a closet tip that I'm famous for. I figured this out years ago, and it just makes so much sense to me. It doesn't matter which way you do it, but just have one shoe pointing in one direction and the other shoe pointing in the other direction. Your shoes stay much better organized that way, and you get an extra pair per shelf.

DAY 20

GREEN

BEAUTY TIP

DID MICHELANGELO KNOW ABOUT THIS? When getting a haircut, approach your hair as if it's part of a sculpture. Make sure your hairdresser looks at the whole you standing up before he or she cuts your hair, taking into consideration how it balances with your whole body. Usually people get their hair cut focusing only on how they look from the shoulders up. They are then shocked when they stand up and don't quite know why it doesn't look right. I learned this tip from a hairdresser years ago who was actually a sculptor. When he did this to me, it made so much sense. I've made sure that every person who cuts my hair since then does the exact same thing. It's the same principle as having a doctor who looks at the whole of you rather than just a specialist who looks at only one part of you.

SPA ON A BUDGET

HAVE YOUR VACATION IN YOUR HOMETOWN. This is a great way to save money. Being a mother helped me figure this one out. When you have children you end up seeing things in your city that you've never seen before. Not just children's activities, but sights. All of a sudden I realized that here I am in Los Angeles, a place that people save a lot of money to come and visit, and there are things here I've never seen. I'm sure that everybody has something they haven't seen in their hometown. A great way to feel like you're on vacation is to appreciate where you live as though you're seeing it for the first time.

TOTAL HEALTH FAKEOVER

IT'S A QUESTION OF BALANCE. When I was on *Taxi*, I got to see myself every single week on television. Now I get to see myself again because the show is on Nick at Nite. I look back on those years, and I realize that one thing I really did learn over the five seasons is how to dress according to proportion. There were times on that show when I was at my thinnest, and I didn't care what I wore. I actually looked sloppy and unbalanced because I thought I could get away with it. The truth is you must always be conscious of proportions and lines. Don't wear anything blocky that cuts you off at the waist if you really are trying to create the illusion of looking taller and thinner. Don't make the mistake of thinking that big, baggy clothes make you look thinner because you're shrinking behind them. Men might be able to get away with that more than women. Women have breasts, and this creates a shelf that everything falls from, actu-

DAY 20

GREEN

197

ally making women look a lot bigger than they are. We all know that black is slenderizing, but sometimes the color black can suck the life right out of your skin. So be very careful not to wear black without any other color someplace else, especially if you have blue or green eyes. You're always going to look healthier if you find a color that matches the color of your eyes.

Menu

DAY 20

On Rising: 6 ounces of fruit juice or 1 piece of seasonal fruit

Breakfast: (2 hours after fruit) Cereal with ¾ cup Rice Dream

Lunch: Quick & Easy Pasta

Snack: Quick Bean Guacamole and Chips

Dinner: Salad in a Bag, Grilled Salmon and Asparagus

Quick & Easy Pasta — Lunch

SERVES 4

1 red onion, sliced
3 cloves garlic, sliced
2 tablespoons olive oil
2 teaspoons crushed red pepper flakes
1 20-ounce can Italian plum tomatoes, drained
1 pound box of linguine
¼ cup minced fresh parsley
Salt and pepper

Sauté the onions and garlic in olive oil over low heat until the onion is wilted. Mix in the pepper flakes and tomatoes. Simmer to thicken for 10 minutes, stirring frequently. Meanwhile, cook the pasta *al dente* in 3 quarts of rapidly boiling water. Drain and transfer to a large pasta bowl. Top with the tomato sauce and parsley and toss to mix thoroughly. Add salt and pepper to taste.

DAY 20

GREEN

Quick Bean Guacamole — Snack

YIELDS 2½ CUPS

1 15-ounce can organic navy or Great Northern beans, drained
1 ripe avocado, scooped out in chunks
¾ cup bottled salsa (mild or hot, according to taste)
1 to 2 tablespoons lime juice
Salt to taste
3 tablespoons finely chopped fresh cilantro for garnish
No-oil corn chips

Place the beans, avocado, salsa, and 1 tablespoon of the lime juice in a food processor. Pulse just enough to create a coarse puree. Add extra lime juice and salt to taste. Transfer to a small serving bowl and garnish with cilantro. Serve with the no-oil corn chips.

Salad in a Bag — Dinner

2 cups mixed greens
½ tomato, sliced or chopped
¼ cucumber, sliced
¼ teaspoon olive oil
½ teaspoon red wine vinegar
Salt and pepper

DAY 20

GREEN

Put the mixed greens into a plastic vegetable bag from the grocery store. Add the tomato, cucumber, olive oil, vinegar, salt, and pepper. Blow up the bag with a couple puffs of air. Shake and serve.

Grilled Salmon and Asparagus — Dinner

SERVES 1

2 shallots, chopped
Juice of 2 limes
1 clove garlic, minced
3 sprigs rosemary, off the stem
8-to-10 ounce salmon fillet
4 to 6 asparagus stalks
Olive oil

In a small bowl, combine the shallots, lime juice, garlic, and rosemary. Let the salmon marinate in the lime mixture for 20 to 30 minutes. Grill approximately 7 minutes on each side. Lightly brush the asparagus with olive oil and grill 2 to 4 minutes on each side.

DAY 20

GREEN

DAY 21

GREEN WEEK

MOTIVATIONAL TIP

JUST REWARDS. As we move toward the final week of this program, let's try not to think of the reward we're going to give ourselves at the end as a food reward. Let's not say, "I can't wait to go pig out after this." Let's start thinking of "reward" not in terms of food, but in terms of little things that might improve our lives. Let's think about a new piece of clothing or furniture, or a manicure and a pedicure or a massage or something indulgent. A great new piece of exercise equipment, some new running shoes, anything that's going to improve the quality of our life over that food reward that we got so often as children. I'm really trying to make it a point as a mother never to give my children food as a reward. If they fall and hurt themselves, I never offer a cookie as a Band-Aid. I know that that's how I grew up, and it's still an automatic response to want to soothe myself anytime something is not 100 percent right. Why not indulge yourself with twenty minutes of fun phone calls to friends? Whatever turns you on besides food is what you should go for.

EXERCISE TIP

IF THE SHOE FITS . . . In any exercise program, good shoes are a must. Replace them every three to six months, depending on how much you work out. If you can't find the style that you like because it's been discontinued, spend the time in the store trying to find a new style that works for you. Make sure your shoes are comfortable because it all starts with your feet. Just find one that fits and makes you want to move. And remember, you should always donate your old shoes to a worthy cause.

FOOD TIP

TABLE FOR TWO. Today we're going to try to turn somebody else on to the program, so invite a friend over for lunch or dinner. The best way to learn is to teach, so teach your friend something about the way you've been eating and discover how much you've learned.

ORGANIZATIONAL TIP

HAVE HANGERS, WILL TRAVEL. Aim to have all of the hangers in your closet exactly alike. Now, I know that sounds complicated but it really isn't. You can buy hangers at a very cheap rate. You can buy them in bulk from a display company. Look in the Yellow Pages. Or start collecting hangers. It's amazing how organized your closet will look and how much better your clothes will slide on the bar when all of the hangers are alike. Start thinking about replacing them a little bit at a time or all at once. I'm so famous for my closets that I've started giving people a gift of reorganizing theirs. One time for Burt Reynolds's birthday I took my whole team of friends over to his house, and we secretly reorganized his closet. His housekeeper told me that as soon as he walked in, he said, "Marilu's been here!"

BEAUTY TIP

ORGANIZE YOUR CLOSET AND BEAUTIFY YOUR FRIENDS. While we're still in our closets, pay attention to what styles you always reach for. There are things that make you feel like you really look good—but see how many things in your closet don't have that effect. Years ago my family decided to do recycled Christmas presents to save money. We decided to give something we no longer needed, but hopefully another person did. There are eight women in my family. So I started making piles of all the things that I had in my closet that would really look good on somebody else. One thing I noticed as I made these piles is that each of the women I was talking about had a certain style. They had a definite look to them that helped me determine which person should get which article of clothing. It was all based on what looked good on that individual body type. I know from experience, from seeing myself so many different ways as different characters, that there are certain styles that just do not look good on me. When they hang in my closet for a long time and I haven't worn them, I always give them away to somebody that I know they will look great on. So, start making a pile of all those things in your closet that you know you're never going to wear but might look good on somebody else and plan to swap or give them away. (Maybe at the final night's party.)

SPA ON A BUDGET TIP

FIGHTS CAVITIES *AND* ZITS. Since we're spending so much time in our closet, I don't want to give you some other assignment that seems too difficult. Here's a little tip for the future. If you ever get a zit, something to do in a pinch is to put a little toothpaste on it to dry it out. Tea tree oil is also great. If you've bought a bottle by now, know that you can dip a Q-Tip in it and put it on a zit and it will magically go away overnight.

TOTAL HEALTH FAKEOVER

ADULT "TIME OUT." Naps should not be just for kids. I don't know if you're going to be able to take a nap today or not, but at least give yourself a little adult time-out. Not to punish yourself but rather to reward yourself for working so hard. Maybe you just need a little ten-minute break to refresh yourself in the middle of the day. Relax, read, think about something else, watch TV, or better yet, listen to Mozart. (Great for the brain cells!) Find a little ten-minute meditation somewhere in your day to sort of cool out. Think of it as a therapeutic adult time-out.

Menu

DAY 21

Breakfast: An all-fruit morning—fruit plate with mixed cantaloupe and honeydew melons (about 2 cups)

Lunch: "I Do" Pasta

Dinner: Border Grill Sea Bass Veracruzana with Steamed Green Beans

"I Do" Pasta—Lunch

SERVES 4

My husband, Rob, and I got married in Italy, and this is the pasta we ate the night before our wedding.

1 large head broccoli
1 pound pasta shells
4 tablespoons olive oil
1–2 large cloves garlic
Crushed red pepper (cayenne) to taste, optional
Salt and pepper to taste

Boil water in a large pasta pot. Cut up 1 head of broccoli (including stems) into small to medium chunks and florets. When the water starts to boil, add the stem chunks, then add the florets. Add the shells and boil 9 to 12 minutes (or use the directions on the pasta box). Remember that the pasta and the broccoli are in the same pot.

In a 10-inch frying pan, combine the olive oil, garlic (I like to press it, some prefer to slice or mince), and red pepper.

When the pasta and broccoli are cooked, strain them in a colander (with small holes—you don't want the cooked broccoli to go to waste). Return the pasta and broccoli to the pot.

Start cooking the oil and garlic over a very low flame. Stir it up so that the garlic is evenly spread out. You want the garlic to get hot, but *don't let it turn brown!* If you do, it will taste bitter and you will have to start again. When it starts to sizzle, pour it over the pasta and broccoli. With a wooden spoon, mix the oil and the pasta. Add salt and pepper to taste.

You will notice that the broccoli and oil form a sauce, and the stems are chunky broccoli treats. The shells scoop up the sauce. Enjoy!

DAY 21

GREEN

Border Grill Sea Bass Veracruzana — Dinner

SERVES 4

This recipe is one of the most popular dishes at Border Grill, a restaurant owned by the Two Hot Tamales, Susan Feniger and Mary Sue Milliken. Susan is a friend of mine, and this is one of my favorite dishes she makes. Border Grill uses the freshest fish available, and a favorite is sea bass, because it sears well in the pan, cooks evenly without flaking, and doesn't overcook easily, which makes it a good choice for a party. The key to this dish is to get the searing pan very hot and caramelize the fish, then quickly fry the vegetable garnish and finish it all with a short simmer.

> 3 tablespoons olive oil
> 1½ pounds skinless, boneless sea bass, or other firm-fleshed fresh fish, cut into 4 portions
> Salt and freshly ground black pepper
> 1 small yellow onion, peeled and thinly sliced
> 2 cloves garlic, peeled and minced
> 2–3 jalapeños, stemmed and sliced in ½-inch disks
> ½ lime, cut in eighths
> 1 tomato, cored, seeded, and cut in strips
> ½ bunch fresh oregano leaves, washed and roughly chopped
> ½ cup white wine
> ¾ cup fish stock or clam juice
> 1 pound steamed green beans

DAY 21

GREEN

Heat one very large or two medium-sized sauté pans over medium heat for a minute, then add olive oil. When sizzling, add the fish fillets seasoned with salt and pepper,

207

flesh side down, and turn the heat to very high. Sear the fillets until golden brown and flip to sear on the other side. Remove the fillets from the pan and reserve on a rack over a plate to catch the juices. Return the pan (or pans) to the heat, add the onion, and cook over high heat for 2 to 3 minutes, stirring often. Add the garlic, jalapeño slices, lime wedges, tomato, and oregano and sauté briskly 1 minute more. Add the white wine and reduce by half. Add the fish stock and bring to a boil. Reduce to a simmer and return the fish fillets along with the juices to the pan. Finish cooking, covered, about 1 to 3 minutes, depending on the thickness of the fillets. Taste the broth and adjust the seasoning, then serve immediately in soup plates with a generous puddle of broth and a garnish of vegetables. Serve with steamed green beans.

Susan Feniger and Mary Sue Milliken
Border Grill, Los Angeles

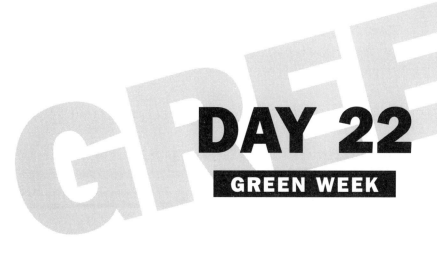

DAY 22

GREEN WEEK

MOTIVATIONAL TIP

GIVE ME A G! Today, as an experiment, try being enthusiastic about everything you do. Try gusto. That little bit of extra energy will dazzle the people you deal with and help inspire their own energy as well. I have never seen this fail. People are so susceptible to another person's mood, because most people wait to see how someone else feels about something. Today you be the one who initiates joy. I'm not saying to do this in a fake or transparent way. But if you're the type who usually waits to read another person's mood, try being the cheerleader for a change and watch what happens.

EXERCISE TIP

DO AN EXERCISE ACTIVITY WITH YOUR KIDS. My kids and I have so much fun together, dancing around the house or playing "It" or doing anything that's going to make us play and sweat at the same time. They don't realize we're exercising. They think they're just playing with Mommy. I don't realize I'm exercising until it's all over and I've gotten my ten- to twenty-minute workout. If you don't have children, maybe you can play with your nieces and nephews.

FOOD TIP

WHEN IN DOUBT, EAT THE CENTERPIECE. Avoid dangerous foods at occasions like picnics and holiday parties. Instead, think about the items that you usually have on those occasions and start thinking of healthy substitutes. You don't have to really give up the dishes that you like to eat. You just have to change some of the ingredients. If you're going to a party where you think they're not going to have anything healthy, make sure that you eat something healthy before you go. There's almost always something that you can eat. You just have to be crafty about figuring out the food that's in front of you. I was in Mississippi performing at a benefit recently, and during a cocktail party there were many things on the buffet table that I couldn't eat. Almost every single thing was made with cream, cheese, or butter. But I noticed that the table decorations were all fresh vegetables. So I sat there eating the centerpiece. Everybody got a big kick out of it. The next day I felt a lot better than I would have had I indulged in all those things that I know take energy from me and clog my nose.

ORGANIZATIONAL TIP

ALWAYS A JACKET, NEVER AN OUTFIT. We've been cleaning out our closets, and we've been going through everything. If there's a borderline pile of clothes that you're not sure you want to give away but you're not sure you ever want to wear again, do a little trick that I always do. I button the jacket or blouse, or sometimes I hang the hanger in the opposite direction so that I know that these are clothes that I probably haven't used in the last six months. If another six-month period goes by and I still haven't used them because they're hanging with the hanger backwards or they're still buttoned up, then I know I'm probably never going to use them, and I give them away. Make this borderline pile in your closet and really evaluate it. What we're trying to do is clean out our closets to make better use of the space we have in there.

DAY 22

GREEN

BEAUTY TIP

IF YOU LOOK GOOD, FLASH! When you look good, don't just flaunt it, copy it. When you feel you really look your best—great outfit, great haircut, whatever—take a picture of yourself from every angle. I learned this tip from being on movie sets and having my picture taken for continuity. Whenever I look especially put together, I always take a picture to remind myself of what it is that I liked about that outfit and how to duplicate it. I take a picture of my hair when it really looks good (front, back, both sides) so that I can remember how to duplicate that. I've also taken that photograph with me to my hairdresser so she can copy the style as well.

SPA ON A BUDGET

WHAT'S OLD TO YOU MIGHT BE NEW TO ME. Plan a recycle party with your friends. (You can do this on Day 30.) Exchange clothes, makeup, books, tapes, and beauty tips. This will allow you to get more bang for your buck by exchanging items you no longer use but don't want to throw out. You've shopped in your own closet— now try shopping in a friend's. You've got some new ideas in your head about the "new" and improved you, and this is a great way not to spend money trying out some new styles.

TOTAL HEALTH FAKEOVER

THINK OF YOUR FANTASY PERSON. Maybe it's Leonardo DiCaprio, Harrison Ford, Elle MacPherson, an old flame, or in my case, Sting. (And who knows, if that restraining order is ever lifted?) Spend your day as if you have a hot date with that person tonight. Notice how you walk through your day taking care of yourself—the energy in your step, the twinkle in your eyes, how every cell in your body stands at attention. Wouldn't it be great if we could always feel that vibrant?

Menu

DAY 22

On Rising: 6 ounces of fruit juice or 1 piece of seasonal fruit

Breakfast: (2 hours after fruit) Maggie Fountain's Tofu Scrambler

Lunch: Chopped Vegetable Salad, Red and White Soup

Dinner: Maggie Fountain's Gourmet Pizza

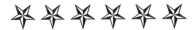

Maggie Fountain's Tofu Scrambler — Breakfast

SERVES 1

DAY 22

GREEN

Maggie Fountain is one of the great success stories of someone who went on this program and completely changed her health and her body. She's a fabulous cook and contributed some tasty recipes for this book.

1 small onion, chopped
½ package firm or extra firm tofu (low-fat tofu is a better choice)
½ cup salsa, hot or mild

Sauté the onion in a pan lightly sprayed with olive oil. Crumble in the tofu and stir it well. Add your sauce of choice and stir. This will take on the consistency of scrambled eggs.

Chopped Vegetable Salad — Lunch

SERVES 4 TO 6

2 cloves garlic, minced
½ cup olive oil
2 beefsteak tomatoes, sliced thick
1 bunch asparagus, ends cleaned
1 large green bell pepper, top and bottom sliced off
2 ears corn on the cob, shucked
3 large carrots, peeled and sliced thick lengthwise
¼ pound fresh green beans, ends trimmed
Salt and freshly ground black pepper
3 tablespoons balsamic vinegar
1 tablespoon Dijon mustard
1 head Romaine lettuce, washed and shredded

In a large bowl, place the garlic and half of the olive oil. Add all the vegetables except the lettuce and season with salt and freshly ground black pepper. Grill the vegetables over medium heat and set aside.

Chop all the vegetables into medium-sized pieces just before serving. To make the vinaigrette, in a small bowl, whisk the balsamic vinegar, Dijon mustard, and remaining olive oil until blended. Add the vinaigrette to the grilled vegetables and place on top of the shredded romaine lettuce.

DAY 22

GREEN

Red and White Soup — Lunch

SERVES 6

4 cups instant vegetable broth or water

1 clove garlic, minced

1 medium onion, chopped

2 medium carrots, chopped

1 head cauliflower, separated into florets

1 cup 1% soy milk

Sea salt and freshly ground black pepper to taste

½ cup salsa, drained

In a large saucepan, combine the broth, garlic, onion, carrots, and cauliflower. Cook over moderate heat for 15 minutes, or until the cauliflower is tender but still firm. With a slotted spoon, remove most of the cauliflower mixture to a blender or food processor, in two batches if necessary. Add the soy milk and puree until smooth, then return to the saucepan. Season with salt and pepper to taste. Rinse the blender container and puree the salsa until smooth. To serve, ladle the soup into bowls and top with a swirl of salsa puree.

DAY 22

GREEN

Maggie Fountain's Gourmet Pizza — Dinner

Who said pizza has to have cheese?

1 teaspoon olive oil
1 ready-to-cook pizza crust
Pizza sauce (read your label—you don't want chemicals or sweeteners)

Toppings

Chopped onions
Garlic
Red, yellow, or green peppers
Mushrooms
Sun-dried tomatoes

Preheat the oven to 400 degrees. Sauté the toppings in the olive oil until tender. Cover the pizza shell with sauce and add the toppings. Garnish with oregano, sweet basil, and rosemary. Add soy cheese if you wish. Bake 20 minutes, or until the crust is crisp.

DAY 22

GREEN

215

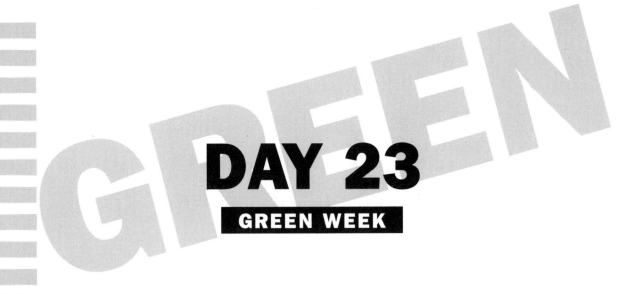

DAY 23

GREEN WEEK

MOTIVATIONAL TIP

HEALTHY SAVINGS ACCOUNT. In the next few weeks, you're going to be shopping on your own. Every time you want to buy something unhealthy to eat, price it and put that money somewhere. Let it accumulate. Not only will you be working toward a healthy goal, you'll have a lot of money to spend on yourself too! When I quit smoking, I tried this technique. When I saw how much money I was saving, it was one of the things that kept me from smoking.

EXERCISE TIP

STRENGTHEN YOUR FUNNY BONE. Exercise your sense of humor. Find the humor in everything that happens today. If all else fails, read today's beauty tip.

FOOD TIP

DON'T START EATING LUNCH UNTIL YOU'VE FINISHED BREAKFAST. Don't eat your next meal until you feel resolved from your last meal. You're starting to get more complicated foods now—more legumes, snacks, and desserts. If something is not agreeing with you or taking a little longer to digest than usual, don't eat the next thing on the list just because it's time for your next meal.

ORGANIZATIONAL TIP

A CLOTHES NOTEBOOK. I get so stressed when it comes to putting outfits together and accessorizing them that I had to start keeping a clothes notebook to help me remember what pieces go together. I grew up wearing a school uniform, so I never got the hang of ensemble dressing. To help me remember what I wore to a special occasion or on a talk show, I keep a notebook of each part of the outfit. This has also been a great way to plan outfits for a trip because I actually have a checklist of everything I need to pack. This cuts down on the number of outfits because I can take some basics and use accessories to make them look different.

BEAUTY TIP

AND NOW HAIR TIPS FROM DAVID! These tips came to me from David Evangelista. He is a funny and talented hairdresser to the stars. He is often seen on *Rosie O'Donnell*, as she is one of his clients. David always exercises his sense of humor.

David's Hair Tips

- To get volume, think of your head as the field of dreams, your hair as the grass, and your fingers as the hoe. If you build volume, they will come! Caution: contrary to popular belief, dragon lady nails do not make good hoes!

- When scrunching your hair, squeeze it as hard as you can, while warming it with the dryer. Squeeze 'til you wheeze! Then stop. We don't need to be fainting, ladies.

- There's a difference between highlights and fry-lights. Don't look like you've been sitting under a red lamp in the bin with McDonald's French fries.

- Frosting is for cupcakes. Enough said.

- When using a curling iron, hold a comb underneath to protect your scalp from burning. Nothing's worse than having a loved one walk in on your beauty routine and ask, "Mmm! Whatcha cooking?"

217

- If someone tries to talk you into a wedge haircut, tell them, "Wedges make good shoes, they can hold a door open, and it's a nice shape for cheese; but not on *my* head, thank you!"

- When choosing a hairstylist, if she's got a big beehive and a Hitler mustache, chances are she isn't auditioning to be a B-52's backup singer. She thinks that look works! Turn and run as fast as you can.

- Short on top, long layers in the back is not pretty. You can't have your short-hair cake and try to eat your long-hair cake too! It sounds gross, but it's true!

- You know you've given yourself a bad color job when the next morning your husband says, "Honey, when did we get tie-dyed sheets?"

- If you want to have shinier hair, rule out eggs, mayonnaise, and beer. They don't really make your hair any shinier than commercial products, but they will make your head smell like a Caesar salad.

- You like French twists? So do I, but make sure they're in proportion to your head. Otherwise, you'll look like a human Q-Tip.

SPA ON A BUDGET TIP

CUSTOM-MAKE YOUR OWN CLOTHES. Make friends with a tailor or dry cleaner. Have your clothes updated by shortening a skirt, changing the buttons on a blazer, or dying an item a current color. Take things in as you shrink in size. Your clothes will look more expensive for less money if they really fit you.

DAY 23

GREEN

TOTAL HEALTH FAKEOVER

INDULGE YOURSELF. Read old love letters or diaries, or look at old pictures. This will put you in a better mood because you feel nostalgic about times past or because you know you're in a better place now.

Menu

DAY 23

On Rising: 6 ounces of fruit juice or 1 piece of seasonal fruit

Breakfast: (2 hours after rising) Nicky's Favorite Oatmeal

Lunch: East-West Egg Salad

Dinner: My Favorite Tuna from Maple Drive Restaurant

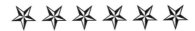

Nicky's Favorite Oatmeal — Breakfast

SERVES 1

DAY 23

GREEN

½ cup oatmeal (quick)
¾ cup boiling water
½ teaspoon maple syrup

Put the oatmeal in a bowl, add the boiling water, and drizzle with the maple syrup.

219

East-West Egg Salad—Lunch

SERVES 4

1 cup steamed tofu, mashed (tofu may be steamed in a vegetable steamer basket over boiling water)
2 hard-boiled egg whites, chopped
½ cup Nayonaise
½ cup chopped bok choy or steamed green beans
½ cup crumbled nori, or more to taste
1 tablespoon gomasio or sesame seeds
1 teaspoon tamari
½ cup chopped water chestnuts, optional
Dried crushed red pepper, optional

Combine all the ingredients until well mixed. Serve with rice cakes, in pita bread, or on a bed of fresh spinach and sprouts.

DAY 23

GREEN

Recipe

My Favorite Tuna from Maple Drive Restaurant—Dinner

SERVES 2

This is my very favorite dish from Maple Drive Restaurant in Beverly Hills.

2 6-ounce portions of freshest, highest-grade 1- to 1½-inch-thick tuna

2½ tablespoons olive oil

Coarsly ground black pepper

3 large handfuls of cleaned spinach leaves

Salt

½ cup julienned scallions

1 cup julienned shiitake mushrooms (stems removed)

Japanese vinaigrette (see following recipe)

Twenty minutes before cooking, rub the tuna with ½ tablespoon olive oil and season generously with black pepper. In a non-stick skillet, sauté the spinach in 1 tablespoon olive oil until lightly cooked. Divide onto 2 plates. Heat a cast iron skillet until very hot. Season the marinated tuna with salt and sear for 2 minutes on each side. Remove and place on top of the spinach.

In a non-stick skillet, sauté the scallions and shiitakes together in 1 tablespoon olive oil until lightly cooked. Place on top of tuna. Pour a little Japanese vinaigrette on and around the tuna. Serve at once.

Leonard Schwartz
Maple Drive Restaurant, Los Angeles

Japanese Vinaigrette — Dinner

MAKES 1 CUP

This recipe works very well as a marinade for shrimp, chicken, and fish, especially tuna, bass, scallops, and mahimahi. It is also a good accompaniment to salads with daikon, daikon sprouts, cucumber, carrot, celery, and watercress. Finally, it makes a delicious dipping sauce for tuna, halibut, or yellowtail sashimi.

- ½ cup peanut oil
- 2 tablespoons soy sauce
- 1 tablespoon Oriental sesame oil
- 2 tablespoons rice wine vinegar
- ½ tablespoon freshly squeezed lemon juice
- ½ tablespoon freshly squeezed lime juice
- 2 tablespoons barley malt
- 2 tablespoons minced, peeled fresh ginger (start with 3 walnut-size pieces)
- ¼ teaspoon minced garlic
- 1 teaspoon minced onion
- 1 teaspoon minced shallots
- ½ teaspoon drained prepared horseradish or freshly grated horseradish
- ¼ teaspoon wasabi powder

DAY 23

GREEN

Whisk together all the liquid ingredients. Place the remaining ingredients in the bowl of a food processor fitted with the steel knife or a blender jar, and add half the liquid ingredients. Process or blend well. Whisk this sauce into the other half of the liquid ingredients, then strain the sauce through a fine sieve. Store refrigerated.

Leonard Schwartz
Maple Drive Restaurant, Los Angeles

DAY 24

YELLOW WEEK KITCHEN LIST

Everything you will need for Yellow Week's menus

Check your kitchen for what you already have. Check recipes for amounts.

Vegetables
Artichoke hearts, canned
Asparagus
Bamboo shoots
Bell pepper: red, green
Bok choy
Broccoli
Cabbage: red and white
Carrots
Celery
Cremini mushrooms
Cucumbers
Garlic, fresh
Green beans
Leeks
Mixed greens
Onion: yellow or white
Peas, frozen
Romaine lettuce

Scallions
Shiitake mushrooms
Spinach
Tomatoes, fresh
Tomatoes, organic plum, canned
Tomatoes with basil, canned

Protein
Anchovies
Eggs
Halibut steaks
Salmon fillets
Tuna, canned in water
Tuna fillets

Fruits & Juices
Juices of choice
Lemon

Lemon juice
Pineapple chunks
Pineapple-coconut juice
Raisins
Seasonal fruits

Grains, Breads, Pasta
Buckwheat mix
Crostini or Italian bread
Croutons
English muffins
Flourless whole-grain bread
Fusilli pasta
Oat bran
Oatmeal
Organic artichoke flour
    angel hair pasta
Pasta of your choice
    (dinner, Day 24)

223

Spanish-style brown rice
  mix
Stale whole wheat bread
  (dessert, Day 28)
Udon noodles
Whole wheat baking mix
  (non-dairy)
Whole wheat pastry flour

Spices

Allspice
Baking powder
Basil, fresh
Black pepper
Chives, fresh
Cinnamon
Crushed red pepper flakes
Dill, fresh
Fine herb seasoning
Ginger root
Hawaiian salt
Italian seasoning
Lemon pepper
Nutmeg
Oregano, fresh
Parsley, fresh
Poppy seeds
Sea salt
Sesame seeds
Vanilla extract

Legumes

Garbanzos (chickpeas)
Lentils
Split peas: green and
  yellow

Miscellaneous

Almond or tahini butter
Almonds, sliced
Balsamic vinegar
Barley malt
Bragg's Liquid Aminos
Canola oil
Coconut milk
Crispy brown rice cereal
Dijon mustard
Flaked coconut
Graham crackers
Honey
Maple syrup
Miso
Nayonaise
Nori (seaweed)
Peanut butter (smooth
  and chunky)
Peanuts
Red wine vinegar
Rice Dream
Rice syrup
Rice wine

Safflower or vegetable oil
Sliced almonds
Sorghum
Soy American cheese
Soy bacon
Soy cream cheese
Soy ham
Soy margarine
Soy milk
Tofu, cake
Tofu, firm
Soy Parmesan
Soy sauce
Sucanat
Tahini
Tahini butter
Tamari
Toasted sesame oil
Tomato paste
Van's brand waffles (no
  dairy)
Vegetable stock
Walnuts
White wine
White wine vinegar
Worcestershire sauce

DAY 24

YELLOW

MOTIVATIONAL TIP

D.I.F.S. DIET. When I was fifteen years old, I was madly in love with a boy named Sammy. He was really something and I would have done anything for him. So I started a diet for him and I called it my D.I.F.S. (Do It For Sammy) diet. It became my mantra—whenever I started to eat something bad I'd say to myself, "D.I.F.S." Years later, when I started eating like I do now, I thought about my D.I.F.S diet and realized I was still on it, but now it meant "Do It For SELF." In this fourth week, if you've been doing this program for your husband, your kids, or for me, it's time to do it for yourSELF.

EXERCISE TIP

LEARN TO MEDITATE. Exercise your inner being. If you don't have a mantra, try to find a neutral word that you can repeat over and over. It doesn't have to be a long meditation, but take five or ten minutes to tune in to yourself. Meditating is not a time of shutting things out, but rather a time of reflection, acceptance, and letting go.

FOOD TIP

SQUEEZE AND SMELL. To know whether a fruit or vegetable is ripe, ask your grocer. Another tip is to use your sense of touch and smell. Many fruits have been sprayed and/or waxed to look better, but they're often tasteless. Organic fruits and vegetables are not as pretty, but they're much tastier and healthier for you. Do not store any vegetables in the plastic bags that you bring them home in unless you plan on using them right away. They'll rot quicker if you do. If you like your fruit cold, put it in the refrigerator only after it's ripened outside the refrigerator.

ORGANIZATIONAL TIP

GIFTS ON HOLD. Whenever I receive a gift that is a duplicate of something I already have, I save it on the "gift shelf" in my closet. In an emergency situation, I always have something to bring to a last-minute birthday party or as a housewarming gift. If you find something that is a big hit as a gift, buy it in multiples. If there's a book or a toy that your child really loves, buy a few extras for friends' kids and give them when they reach the appropriate age.

BEAUTY TIP

BEAUTY ISN'T ONLY SKIN DEEP. Look into your heart. Find the beauty of the soul. Spend the day reaching out to others and looking at the acts of kindness in others. If you really open yourself up to the love in you and in the people around you, you'll be amazed at how beautiful you can feel inside. All that love will radiate outside.

SPA ON A BUDGET

TRADE YOUR STRENGTHS WITH A FRIEND. If you do something well, trade that service for something that a friend does better than you do. For example, I have two friends, and one makes jewelry and the other cuts hair. They'll exchange one for the other, and both benefit. You don't have to limit yourself to a product, either. I recently had lunch with a friend, and I gave him nutritional advice while he gave me business advice. Maybe there's someone you can exchange carpooling for dog walking services. The list is endless.

DAY 24

YELLOW

TOTAL HEALTH FAKEOVER

SCENTURY 21. Create the illusion of harmony in your environment; buy fresh flowers, light scented candles, put on soothing music. If your environment seems balanced, so do you. This tip worked really well for me when I went to sell my house and had cinnamon potpourri brewing in the kitchen. The first people who saw the house bought it because they said they wanted a house that smelled so good.

Menu

DAY 24

On Rising: 6 ounces fruit juice or 1 piece of fresh fruit

Breakfast: (2 hours after fruit) Van's Brand Waffles (no dairy)

Lunch: Maggie Fountain's Pea Soup

Dinner: Autumn Tomato Bruschetta, Lentil Pasta with Green Beans Italian Style

DAY 24

YELLOW

Maggie Fountain's Pea Soup — Lunch

SERVES 4

1 small onion
1 medium carrot
2 cups green or yellow split peas
6 cups water
Sea salt and pepper to taste

Finely chop the onion and carrot. Combine all the ingredients and simmer, covered, on low heat for 1 to 2 hours.

Autumn Tomato Bruschetta — Dinner

SERVES 2

Chopped garlic to taste
1 tablespoon olive oil
1 large tomato, chopped
Salt to taste
Crostini or other Italian bread

DAY 24

YELLOW

In a small bowl, mix the garlic, oil, and tomato. Sprinkle with salt and put on top of sliced bread. Toasting is optional.

Lentil Pasta — Dinner

SERVES 4

4 cloves garlic
½ teaspoon pepper
¼ cup olive oil
1 bunch asparagus
1 can lentils
1 can tomatoes with basil
¼ teaspoon Italian seasoning
⅛ cup Bragg's Liquid Aminos
⅛ cup white wine
¼ cup basil
1 pound pasta, your choice, cooked

In a large pan, sauté the garlic and pepper in the olive oil. Add the asparagus. Sauté for 2 minutes, then add the lentils, tomatoes, Italian seasoning, and Bragg's. Let simmer. If it gets dry, add white wine. Add the basil and let simmer 5 to 10 minutes. Pour over the cooked pasta of your choice.

Green Beans Italian Style — Dinner

SERVES 4

1 pound tender young green beans
Ground sea salt
2 teaspoons balsamic vinegar
2 tablespoons extra virgin olive oil

Bring lots of water to a boil in a large pot. Trim the ends of the beans and cut or break them in half. Add a pinch of ground rock salt and beans to the water. Cook at a rolling boil for 3 minutes, or until bright green and tender. Drain and rinse in a large bowl of ice water. Drain and pat dry.

Place the green beans in a bowl. Sprinkle with the balsamic vinegar and toss well. Add the olive oil and toss again to thoroughly coat the beans with oil. Serve chilled or at room temperature.

DAY 24

YELLOW

DAY 25

YELLOW WEEK

MOTIVATIONAL TIP

The doctor of the future will give no medicine, but will interest his patients in the care of the human frame, in diet, and in the care and prevention of disease.

—*Thomas A. Edison*

The physician is only nature's assistant.

—*Galen*

Remember to cure the patient as well as the disease.

—*Dr. Alvin Barach*

PREVENTIVE NOT PRESCRIPTIVE. Shouldn't we be doing this now? How long do we have to wait for doctors to recognize that we should be concentrating on prevention? What I'm hoping to accomplish with this program is make people aware of the inner workings of their own bodies. People who become so conscious of their own health that they will be able to really help their doctors help them. We will feel so well trained in taking care of ourselves that we will be able to feel the symptoms and the early signs of disease as soon as they happen. We will help our doctors become nature's assistants.

DAY 25

YELLOW

EXERCISE TIP

"**TRAVELEROBICS.**" Consider exercise as part of your next vacation or weekend trip. Most people think of vacations as a time to pig out and lie still. Instead, check the local paper or magazines and look for athletic opportunities. At least take advantage of the health club that might be in your hotel or nearby. You will be just as rested when you come home, if not more so. How many times have we come home from a vacation exhausted? You will be healthier and rejuvenated, and you won't need a vacation when you get back. Plus you won't have to lose the ten pounds you would have gained.

FOOD TIP

LET FOOD BE YOUR MEDICINE AND MEDICINE BE YOUR FOOD. There's so much power in every single thing we eat. At this point in the program, we should understand how different foods affect us (whether or not we get energy from them, or if they make us sleepy in a good way). Certain foods can lower our cholesterol, boost our immune systems, or alleviate the symptoms of disease. We should respect the energy in food and not let it take energy away from us.

ORGANIZATIONAL TIP

SHARE THE HEALTH! Add natural products to your gift giving. Next time you go to the health food store and there's a product that you really like, maybe someone in your life would like it as well. Put it on your gift shelf. Also, for a child's birthday gift, how about adding a sugar-free treat to the bowl? Kids don't realize how sweet non-sugar treats are. A lot of times they're really surprised at my son's school when I bring something in and it's just as sweet as the candy made with refined sugar they're used to. This is a good way to turn children and their parents on to health.

DAY 25

YELLOW

BEAUTY TIP

I COULD HAVE DANCED ALL NIGHT. Have at least one pair of dressy shoes that are comfortable. Nothing will make you look less healthy and more miserable than uncomfortable shoes. My outfit always starts with the shoes that will go with what I'll be doing that night. (If I'm standing at a cocktail party, for example, I won't wear tight shoes.) I've learned the hard way not to torture myself by wearing uncomfortable shoes that might look good with an outfit but make me absolutely miserable.

SPA ON A BUDGET

BUY THE TREND. Every season of fashion has its list of "must-haves." According to my friend Sharon Feldstein, stylist to the stars, nothing will make you feel more current than buying one of them in whatever price range you can afford or want to spend. For example, if a certain color is "in," I'll buy an item in a shade of that color that looks good on me just so that I'll feel as if I know what's going on. I won't necessarily buy a cashmere sweater, but I'll buy a ten-dollar scarf. If you don't give yourself something new even on the smallest level, you'll never feel like you're a part of the modern world. For a small amount of money, you can still look current.

TOTAL HEALTH FAKEOVER

MEET ME AT THE MALL. Go to the food court at the mall and watch how badly people are eating. Sodas, pizzas, burgers, sugary desserts, nachos—and all the different smells—assault you as you walk by all the high-fat, high-sugar foods. Commend yourself on your healthy intentions. You'll feel you have the upper hand on your future if you're no longer a slave to mass appeal.

DAY 25

YELLOW

Menu

DAY 25

Breakfast: All-fruit breakfast, 2 or 3 pieces from the proper list

Lunch: My Favorite Stir-fry

Dinner: Salmon Teriyaki with Spinach and Scallions, Peanut Butter Cookies (2)

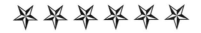

DAY 25

YELLOW

My Favorite Stir-fry — Lunch

SERVES 6

Sauce

3 tablespoons tamari

1 tablespoon toasted sesame oil

½ teaspoon barley malt

¼ cup water

1 teaspoon kuzu (healthy replacement for cornstarch), optional

Stir-fry

2 tablespoons safflower or vegetable oil

3 scallions, thinly sliced

2 medium leeks (white part only), washed and thinly sliced

2 teaspoons fresh ginger root, peeled and minced

3 fresh shiitake mushrooms, thinly sliced

1 red bell pepper, julienned

1 cup bamboo shoots, drained

¼ cup sliced almonds

1½ cups cooked brown rice

1 tablespoon brown rice vinegar

1 head romaine lettuce, washed and leaves separated

In a cup, combine the sauce ingredients and reserve. Heat a wok or large sauté pan over moderately high heat and add the oil, scallions, leeks, and ginger. Stir-fry for about 5 minutes. Add the mushrooms, bell pepper, bamboo shoots, almonds, brown rice, vinegar, and reserved sauce. Cook until heated through. Serve on a bed of lettuce and, if desired, eat by rolling up the rice mixture in the lettuce leaves.

DAY 25

YELLOW

Salmon Teriyaki with Spinach and Scallions — Dinner

SERVES 4

¼ cup rice wine

2 tablespoons soy sauce

2 teaspoons toasted sesame oil

1 teaspoon barley malt

1 tablespoon peeled, minced fresh ginger

1 large clove garlic, minced

2 1½-pound 1¼-inch-thick salmon fillets, skinned

1 teaspoon olive oil

¾ pound fresh spinach, trimmed

10 thin scallions, cut into 2-inch-long julienne

1 tablespoon sesame seeds

Freshly ground black pepper

2 tablespoons minced fresh chives

In a glass dish just large enough to hold the salmon, whisk together the rice wine, soy sauce, sesame oil, barley, ginger, and garlic. Add the fillets and marinate for 30 minutes at room temperature. Turn the fish and marinate for 15 minutes more.

Preheat the oven to 500 degrees. Oil an ovenproof casserole that is just large enough to hold the fish and spinach. Rinse the spinach, but do not dry thoroughly. Place the spinach in the casserole and scatter half of the scallions on top. Remove the fish from the marinade and place over the spinach. Pour the marinade over the fillets. Sprinkle evenly with the remaining scallions, sesame seeds, and pepper. Tightly cover the casserole with foil. Bake until the fish is firm to the touch and not quite opaque in the center, about 15 minutes.

Divide the fish and spinach among 4 heated plates. Spoon some pan juices over the fish if you wish. Sprinkle with a bit more pepper and chives.

Peanut Butter Cookies — Dessert

YIELD: 2 DOZEN

¾ cup peanut butter
½ cup sorghum
¼ cup date sugar
⅓ cup oil
¼ teaspoon sea salt
1 teaspoon vanilla extract
1 cup whole wheat pastry flour

Preheat the oven to 350 degrees. In a large bowl, combine all the ingredients except the flour; gradually mix the flour in. Drop the batter by teaspoonful onto a greased cookie sheet. Flatten each cookie with a fork. Bake 8 to 10 minutes.

DAY 25

YELLOW

DAY 26

YELLOW WEEK

MOTIVATIONAL TIP

IF YOU CAN'T HIDE IT, DECORATE IT. Focus on a body part that you previously hated but is now getting better. Spend the day loving it. Dress for it, celebrate it, work it. It's time to show a little bit of shape, because the good is getting great and the bad is getting better. As I've already told you, my least favorite body part is my middle. If I've been extra-committed to the program, I won't go out and buy a navel ring, but I will tuck in a blouse.

EXERCISE TIP

FITTING IN. Fit is measured in seven ways:

1. Endurance

2. Strength

3. Flexibility

4. Speed

5. Coordination

6. Agility

7. Equilibrium

238

Remember I asked you to evaluate yourself in these areas during Countdown? How do you feel about yourself now?

FOOD TIP

FOOD FOR THOUGHT. Don't be afraid to go to a restaurant, a party, or someone's house for dinner. Ask yourself two questions after you get there, "How hungry am I?" and "What do I feel like eating?" Really answer those questions for yourself. Don't open the menu or start eating until you do. Let your new healthy instincts plan your meals.

ORGANIZATIONAL TIP

CARD SHARK. Build a collection of greeting cards. Don't buy only one card at a time. Buy cards that you like and save them in a small box. This isn't meant to create more clutter. In fact, quite the contrary. It helps save time and clutter. At the very least you'll always have a card for that last-minute occasion.

BEAUTY TIP

WALK, RUN, AND ROLL—SPECIAL EVENT TROUBLESHOOTING. There's usually a lot of nervousness attached to special events, I practice these three little troubleshooting techniques to help get me get through the night. First, I break in my shoes beforehand by wearing them with thick socks. Or I ask someone with bigger feet to walk around in them for a while, like my brother. (Although I think he's beginning to enjoy this too much. Lately he's been asking to break in my dresses, too.) Second, I always make sure that I have two pairs of pantyhose that go with the outfit. Chances are I'm going to run one of them. Third, I always pin the back of my pantyhose to my bra for a nice, long, roll-free look. People tease me about this all the time, but it really helps give a dressy outfit that nice, clean, smooth line. (I don't know why a stocking manufacturer

239

hasn't thought of this. Maybe I'll create my own line.) What you do is you pin the band of the stockings with two large safety pins that can go inside or outside your bra. It pulls the back of your bra down, it gives you a lift in the front, and you don't get that stupid pantyhose roll right across your waist.

SPA ON A BUDGET TIP

SWEAT IS A GREAT VOLUMIZER! I know this sounds a little crazy, but sometimes when I need texture in my hair, I'll wash my hair early. Then I blow it out, set it or do whatever I have to do to it. I will then get on the treadmill and walk just to get a little sweat volume in my hair. I learned this from a hair expert, and it's amazing how much texture you get in your hair from this. You can still take a shower afterwards, of course. It's just that your hair doesn't have that freshly washed softness that needs a lot of product to give it volume. As volumizers go, there's nothing cheaper than sweat.

TOTAL HEALTH FAKEOVER

WALK THE TALK. When I want to foster certain habits in my children or in other people, I try to do it by example and not by lecturing them. If you want your children, your husband, or your friends to be healthy eaters, of course begin with yourself. If you don't want the kids to have chemicals in their food, then get rid of the soda and all the other chemical containing foods in your house. You have to surround yourself with good things. When you're a role model, think of yourself in that role (even if you're faking it for a while).

Menu

DAY 26

On Rising: Fruit juice or 1 piece of fresh fruit

Breakfast: (2 hours after fruit) Piña Colada Muffins (1)

Lunch: TV Guide Tuna

Dinner: Presto Paella, Brown Rice Crispy Treats (2)

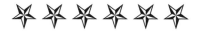

Piña Colada Muffins — Breakfast

YIELDS 8 MUFFINS

1½ cups whole wheat baking mix, non-dairy
2 teaspoons baking powder
½ cup oat bran
½ cup flaked coconut
¼ cup canola oil
1 egg white, beaten
1 cup piña colada (pineapple-coconut) juice
½ cup Rice Dream or soy milk
1 cup pineapple chunks

Preheat the oven to 375 degrees. In a mixing bowl, combine the baking mix, baking powder, oat bran, and ¼ cup of the coconut. Stir in the oil, egg white, piña colada juice, and Rice Dream or soy milk. Gently fold in the pineapple chunks. Spoon the batter into lightly greased muffin tins. Bake for 20 minutes, or until a toothpick inserted in the batter comes out clean. Turn out onto a rack to cool and sprinkle with the remaining coconut while still warm, pressing it in slightly so it adheres.

DAY 26

YELLOW

TV Guide Tuna — Lunch

SERVES 4 TO 6

This is a dish my kids love. We named it TV Guide Tuna because it seems like a recipe you would find there.

> **1 pound cooked fusilli pasta**
> **2 cans tuna fish packed in water, lightly drained**
> **2 tablespoons Nayonaise**
> **1 10-ounce package frozen peas, cooked and drained**
> **Bragg's Liquid Aminos, optional**

Mix the ingredients. Lightly season with Bragg's and serve.

Presto Paella — Dinner

SERVES 2 TO 4

> **1 5-ounce box Spanish-style brown rice mix (Casbah or Near East brands, if possible)**
> **1½ cups cooked chickpeas**
> **2 cups broccoli spears**
> **2 medium carrots, sliced**
> **⅓ cup marinated artichoke hearts**

Prepare the rice mix according to the package directions. While the rice is cooking, add the chickpeas. Place the broccoli in the center of the pan and arrange the sliced carrots around the edge. Cover for about 5 minutes so the vegetables steam. Divide the rice among the plates and top with vegetables. Before serving, garnish with the artichoke hearts.

DAY 26

YELLOW

Brown Rice Crispy Treats—Dessert

SERVES 12

1 box crispy brown rice cereal
1 cup rice syrup
½ cup peanut, almond, or tahini butter
½ cup peanuts, optional

Lightly oil a 9-by-12-inch Pyrex pan. Pour the cereal into a large bowl. In a saucepan, heat the rice syrup over medium-low heat until it bubbles. Add the peanut butter and peanuts. Stir until the rice syrup and peanut butter melt together. Quickly pour over the cereal in the bowl. Mix together with a spatula until the cereal is lightly coated. Transfer the crispy mixture into the Pyrex dish. Press the cereal down and smooth out the top. Let set a bit before cutting into desired pieces. Store covered.

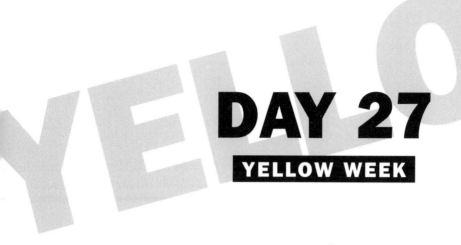

DAY 27
YELLOW WEEK

MOTIVATIONAL TIP

Every education is a kind of inward journey.

—*Vaclav Havel, President of the Czech Republic*

PREPARE YOURSELF WITH KNOWLEDGE. Feeling without knowledge is simply distress. Before this program you may have panicked about what to eat and what to do. But now you know. Now you don't have to feel stressful about it because you've been given the knowledge. You've taken this journey. You're now at a point where you can figure things out for yourselves. Hopefully through the education of this program, you've gone deeper into your inward journey. I always say you only feel panicky if you haven't done your homework. Now you've done your homework, so you don't have to feel panicky.

EXERCISE TIP

ASS GOOD AS IT GETS. Have fun while you tighten those buns. Everyone wants a firm and toned butt. Unfortunately, it is one of the hardest areas to firm. We have to consistently target muscles that are difficult to reach and isolate because we usually exhaust nearby muscles first, such as the quadriceps. If the thought of using conventional glute machines at the gym three times a week sounds painful and boring,

245

consider taking a beginner's ballet class once a week. You'll develop more grace and balance, and those endless pliés will stimulate the fibers in your gluteus to the maximus. You'd be surprised how many dance schools offer beginning ballet for adults. Ballet is great for you men out there who are secure enough with your masculinity and want great buns. However, if this doesn't "sit" well with your Teamster buddies, try basketball. All that jumping gives your rump a pumping. It doesn't target the glutes as well as ballet, though. Compare the backsides of Baryshnikov and Larry Byrd.

FOOD TIP

PASSPORT TO HEALTHY FOODS. Shop the ethnic food aisle. You're going to be grocery shopping on your own next week. You're going to be buying all sorts of things for yourself. A good place to look (and this is in any store, not just a health food store) is the ethnic food aisle. Every ethnicity offers itself to healthy eating, including beans, rice, lentils, tamari, marinades, and spices. You just have to find where the good, healthy food is stocked in your local grocery store.

ORGANIZATIONAL TIP

READY TO GO "THANK-YOU'S." Buy a box of thank-you cards, pre-stamp them, and write your return address. If you keep them handy, the next time you receive a gift or a favor you can immediately write out a nice thank-you note. Some of us have lost the art of writing thank-you notes. It sometimes takes us three weeks to get to it, and by then it has lost some of its impact. If you make it convenient for yourself, you'll do it right away.

BEAUTY TIP

DAY 27

YELLOW

HOW TO DRESS FOR CARNEGIE HALL? *PRACTICE, PRACTICE, PRACTICE.* A way to help yourself de-stress for an event is to have a dress rehearsal. Try on everything, including underwear, hose, shoes, bag, wrap. Experiment with the new hairdo you planned on trying. If it's really an important event, you want to avoid being nervous that night. You don't want to be scrambling at the last minute trying to put things together. (Believe me, I had to learn this the hard way!)

SPA ON A BUDGET TIP

CLOSE CALL. For a really close shave under your arms without any bumps or irritation, use Vaseline. You'll get the closest shave possible. You might ruin a blade, so you're not going to do this every time. But I do this whenever I'm wearing a sleeveless gown on an awards show or special event, or any time I have to show my underarms for a play or a movie.

TOTAL HEALTH FAKEOVER

MIRROR, MIRROR ON THE WALL—*PART II!* Remember in week one we looked in our thin mirror and said we were going to pretend we're that person and not use it as an excuse to eat? Well, now you could even look in the *fat* mirror in your house, and walk, talk, dress, and eat like the lean, healthy person you are. In other words, don't ever let what you think you see in the mirror affect the inner, healthy you. Don't let images derail you.

Menu

DAY 27

On Rising: Fruit juice or 1 piece of fresh fruit

Breakfast: (2 hours after fruit) Egg White Omelet with
Soy Cream Cheese and Vanilla and Basil

Lunch: Jazzy Niçoise

Dinner: Open Sesame Noodles, Crunchy Crisps (2)

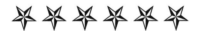

Egg White Omelet with Soy Cream Cheese and Vanilla and Basil — Breakfast

SERVES 1

3 egg whites
Splash of vanilla
1 leaf fresh basil, chopped, or ⅛ teaspoon dried basil
1 tablespoon soy cream cheese

DAY 27

YELLOW

Beat the egg whites with the vanilla and basil and place in a Teflon pan or a lightly canola oil–sprayed non-Teflon pan over high heat. When the omelet is almost set, place soy cream cheese on one side and fold over.

Jazzy Nicoise — Lunch

SERVES 4

⅓ cup olive oil
1 large onion, sliced
½ teaspoon salt
¼ teaspoon white pepper
3 tomatoes, peeled, seeded, and diced
1 bunch oregano, leaves only, chopped
½ cup small green olives, with pits
1½ tablespoons chopped capers, with juice
4 6-ounce tuna fillets
Salt and white pepper to taste
Mixed greens

Heat 3 tablespoons of the oil in a medium skillet over moderate heat. Cook the onion with the salt until soft, about 10 minutes. Combine the pepper, tomatoes, oregano, and olives in a bowl. Add the cooked onion and chill.

Season the tuna all over with salt and pepper. Cook on a very hot, clean grill, about 3 minutes per side. The inside should be bright pink. Transfer to a platter and chill. To serve, arrange the fillets on individual plates. Spoon over the tomato and olive compote and serve cold over mixed greens.

DAY 27

YELLOW

Open Sesame Noodles — Dinner

SERVES 4

¼ cup Nayonaise

1 teaspoon lemon juice

1½ tablespoons miso

2 or 3 drops chili oil (more if you like it spicy)

3 ounces udon noodles, broken into 3-inch pieces, cooked and cooled

½ cup Bragg's Liquid Aminos

1 large tomato, diced

1 large cucumber, sliced

¼ cup sesame seeds

1 celery stalk, sliced

¼ cup chopped parsley

In a large bowl, whisk together the Nayonaise, lemon juice, miso, and chili oil. Add the udon noodles, Bragg's, tomato, cucumber, sesame seeds, celery, and parsley and toss to coat with the dressing. If desired, serve on individual lettuce leaves.

DAY 27

YELLOW

Crunchy Crisps — Dessert

YIELDS 16 PIECES

½ **cup chunky peanut butter**
½ **cup honey or maple syrup**
½ **teaspoon vanilla extract**
½ **teaspoon cinnamon**
2 **cups crispy brown rice cereal**

In a large bowl, mix the peanut butter, honey, vanilla, and cinnamon until well combined. Add the cereal and fold in gently until evenly coated. Cover and set aside for 20 minutes. Place a dish of water nearby and cover a cookie sheet or plate with waxed paper. With wet hands, squeeze the mixture into walnut-sized balls and place them on the sheet to harden. If desired, roll in shredded coconut or sesame seeds.

DAY 27

YELLOW

251

DAY 28

YELLOW WEEK

MOTIVATIONAL TIP

MEASURE UP. Make an appointment to take your internal measurements again. See how you've improved in the last four weeks. I'm sure that your cholesterol has gone down, and if your blood pressure was high, that probably went down as well.

EXERCISE TIP

FIND YOUR TARGET HEART RATE. I went through this in *Total Health Makeover*. If you want to work out at the low end of your target rate, you need to exercise twice as long. If you want to work out near the maximum of your target heart rate, you can spend less time. So, would you rather get it over with, or would you rather take the scenic route? Either way, each day it's important to do something. Each day is unique, so adjust your exercise to your time needs. To find your target heart rate, subtract your age from 220. That number is the absolute maximum level you should ever work at. Multiply your maximum rate by the percentage you want to work at, somewhere between 60 and 80 percent.

FOOD TIP

UP, UP AND NO WHEY! You don't have to eat unhealthy meals when you fly. You just need to know what to order. There are quite a few healthy meals you can order when you travel. I've been told by the airlines that the healthiest meal you could order is the kosher vegetarian meal because it's absolutely the freshest food. Continental Airlines provides a list of possible meals you can order; they include special meals for diabetics, gluten free, low calorie, low cholesterol and low fat, low sodium, dairy free, Hindu, Moslem, Asian vegetarian, vegan, and lacto-ovo vegetarian. You can order fruit plates, seafood only, children's meals, and infants' meals! Who knew?

ORGANIZATIONAL TIP

SMART PACKING. If you're packing for a trip or you're moving, use some of the packing tips that I've learned. First, stuff your socks in your shoes to keep their shape. Second, save plastic bags from the dry cleaners or ask for extras. You can pack your hanging clothes in them so you won't have to iron your clothes when you get there. It's amazing how much time and energy that saves. Third, roll your sweaters and T-shirts, or pack them completely flat if you need the extra space. This will avoid having to iron them when you get there as well.

BEAUTY TIP

BEAUTY ON CLOUD NINE. A beauty tip while you're on an airplane is to make sure you drink plenty of water, wear a minimal amount of makeup, and keep spraying your face with a light spray bottle of water. Moisturize your face as often as you can, or get a Reviva vitamin E stick and put it on all those little wrinkle spots on your face. Keep your hands well creamed. Take your shoes off periodically and really give your feet a workout while you're on an airplane. Get up and stretch as often as you possibly can. Walk the aisles. You might also want to get one of those little pillows for your neck that you can buy at airport gift shops. They're very inexpensive, and I can't tell you how much they save your neck.

SPA ON A BUDGET

GOOD THINGS COME IN SMALL PACKAGES. You know those small bottles of products in hotels? The hotels expect you to take them with you. Even if you don't like the brands they give you in the hotel, you can recycle the container and fill it with your own stuff for the next time you travel, or save the samples from the hotels and put them in your guest room for guests who may have forgotten their toiletries.

TOTAL HEALTH FAKEOVER

LIVE IN A NEW AGE. Broaden your horizons. Today, think of yourself as younger and experimental or older and more sophisticated. Wear jeans or a suit, a ponytail or a chignon, go to a rock concert or an opera. Playing in another age range will help you appreciate where you've been or where you're going.

Menu

DAY 28

On Rising: 6 ounces fruit juice or 1 piece of seasonal fruit

Breakfast: (2 hours after fruit) Henner McMuffin

Lunch: Miso Broth with Vegetables

Dinner: Rob's Caesar Salad, Josie's Pasta, Special Bread Pudding

Henner McMuffin — Breakfast

SERVES 1

Lightly fried egg white
1 toasted English muffin
1 piece soy cheese
1 piece lightly grilled soy ham or soy bacon

Place the fried egg white on top of the English muffin. Place the soy cheese and soy ham or bacon on top.

Miso Broth with Vegetables — Lunch

SERVES 2

2 cups filtered water
3 shiitake mushrooms, cleaned and sliced
3 cremini mushrooms, cleaned and sliced
¼ cup julienned carrots
¼ cup bok choy (asparagus can be substituted)
¼ cup firm tofu, cut into ½ inch disks
1 scallion, sliced
1 1-inch by 6-inch sheet toasted nori (seaweed), julienned
1 tablespoon miso or to taste

Heat the water in small pot. Add the vegetables and simmer for 2 to 3 minutes. Pour into a bowl over the tofu and garnish with the sliced scallion and toasted nori. (Never put miso into boiling water.) Mix in the miso.

255

DAY 28

YELLOW

Rob's Soy Caesar — Dinner

SERVES 6 TO 8

1 egg yolk
2 small cloves garlic
1 teaspoon Worcestershire sauce
1 teaspoon Dijon mustard
Juice of ½ lemon
4 to 6 anchovy fillets
⅓ cup olive oil
Salt to taste
Freshly ground black pepper to taste
3 heads Romaine lettuce, washed and cut into large pieces
¼ cup soy Parmesan
Croutons, optional

Blend the egg yolk, garlic, Worcestershire, mustard, lemon juice, and anchovies in a food processor; slowly drizzle in the olive oil. Season with salt and pepper. In a large mixing bowl, toss the lettuce with the dressing and sprinkle in the soy Parmesan and more pepper. Serve with croutons if desired.

Josie's Pasta — Dinner

SERVES 4

This recipe is from one of my favorite restaurants in the world!

2 tablespoons extra virgin olive oil
5 cloves garlic, sliced
⅓ cup diced yellow onion
12 basil leaves, rolled and thinly sliced (chiffonade)
1½ tablespoons tomato paste
32-ounce can organic plum tomatoes, drained and sliced
2 teaspoons salt
½ teaspoon crushed red pepper flakes
1 pound organic artichoke flour angel hair pasta

Heat the oil in a skillet and sauté the garlic and onion until lightly browned. Add half the basil and the tomato paste. Continue to cook for 2 more minutes. Add the tomatoes (sliced lengthwise) to the pan. Simmer 10 to 12 minutes and add the salt and red pepper flakes. Cook the angel hair pasta in boiling salted water until it is half done and drain. Add the pasta to the sauce and cook on a low flame until some of the sauce has been absorbed into the pasta. Transfer to a serving bowl, sprinkle the remaining basil on top, and serve.

Louis Lanza
Josie's Restaurant, New York

Special Bread Pudding — Dessert

SERVES 6

8 slices stale whole wheat bread

1 cup soy milk

⅓ cup raisins, optional (better for food combining if you don't use)

3 tablespoons soy margarine

⅔ cup sucanat or honey

1 tablespoon allspice

1 egg white

4 tablespoons soy milk

Pinch of ground nutmeg

Preheat the oven to 350 degrees. Roughly break up the bread and place in a mixing bowl with 1 cup soy milk. Let soak. Add the raisins, margarine, sucanat or honey, and allspice. Beat well. Whisk together the egg white and 4 tablespoons soy milk and add to bread mixture. Turn into a greased shallow ovenproof dish, level the surface, and sprinkle with ground nutmeg. Bake for about 45 minutes, or until set. Serve hot or cold.

DAY 29

MOTIVATIONAL TIP

DON'T WAIT FOR YOUR LIFE TO BEGIN. Whatever it's going to take for you to turn into the fabulous person you know you can be, do it now. If it means going into therapy, if it means losing weight, if it means going on this program all over again, if it means getting rid of some of the deadbeat relationships in your life—whatever it's going to take—you should start to do it as soon as possible. When I was young and wanted to go into therapy, people said to me, "Why do you want to go into therapy? You're so young." And I said, "Because I don't want to wait to be a wise old person. I want to be a wise young person." Don't wait for someone to give you permission to begin your life. Start the rest of your life as soon as possible.

EXERCISE TIP

ID YOUR EXERCISE PERSONALITY. PART II. We did this in Countdown on Day 4. Look again at the different types on page 91. Now that you know which one you are, pick one of the other personalities to try.

FOOD TIP

HALF AND HALF YOUR WAY TO HEALTH. Next week you're going to be choosing food for yourself for the first time after completing this 30-day plan. If you still feel like you need to wean yourself off of overly salty, overly sugared, and overly fatty foods, this is what you should start to do. When you have a bowl of popcorn, make half of it the oily popcorn and half of it air popped. Start mixing French fries with "air" fries. Dilute your juice with water so it isn't so sweet. Find little ways to retrain your palate and/or lower your fat intake.

ORGANIZATIONAL TIP

JUNK PILE WARFARE. As you walk around your house today, take note of any pile of junk that still exists. (Old clothes, mail, stacks of magazines, anything you've been putting off sorting through.) Tackle it once and for all. If there are too many piles to go through, try to do at least one a day or one a week until all the piles are gone. Avoid creating future piles by using "The Box." I have a box that sits in my bathroom on the floor, and anything that's unsightly, I put in this box. As soon as the box fills up, I know that I have to start sorting through it and putting things away.

BEAUTY TIP

LET THE SUNSHINE OUT! Always use a hair product with sunscreen in it. Without it, your hair will definitely lighten whether or not you color it and the oils in your hair will dry out, leaving it dull and lifeless. We all know to protect our skin with sunscreen, but don't forget to put sunscreen on the back of your hands to avoid age spots. If you already have them, it's best to use aloe vera to fade them out. Apply fresh aloe vera on each spot with a Q-Tip.

SPA ON A BUDGET TIP

NOW YOU SEE IT, NOW YOU DON'T. Since I'm so hamper, these three stain removal tips have saved me more than once. If you have a stain or a spot on white clothing, take a Q-Tip and dip it in Clorox and apply it carefully to the troubled area. I've saved so many stained T-shirts this way. The best way to get rid of red wine is with white wine, followed by club soda. And to remove ballpoint pen marks, use hair spray or nail polish remover.

TOTAL HEALTH FAKEOVER TIP

FRIEND MAINTENANCE DAY. Designate one day a month (or one day a week if you have the time) to friend maintenance day. Catch up on phone calls or write letters to old friends or relatives. This is a perfect rainy Sunday morning or afternoon activity. Nothing will put you in a better mood than catching up with old friends.

Menu

DAY 29

Breakfast: Fruit Morning: select 2 pieces of your choice from approved list on page 223

Lunch: "Bacon," Lettuce, and Tomato Sandwich with Rob's Cole Slaw

Dinner: Halibut with Aunt Eunice's Marinade for Everything with Braised Bok Choy, Legal Cheesecake

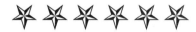

"Bacon," Lettuce, and Tomato Sandwich — Lunch

SERVES 1

2 slices whole grain bread
1 teaspoon Nayonaise
2 leaves lettuce
2 slices tomato
2 slices soy bacon

Toast whole grain bread. Spread on the teaspoon of Nayonaise. Place the lettuce, tomato, and soy bacon on the bread.

Rob's Cole Slaw — Lunch

SERVES 8

¾ head white cabbage, shredded
¼ head red cabbage, shredded
1 large carrot, shredded
½ red pepper, shredded
½ green pepper, shredded
1 large red tomato, shredded
1 cup Nayonaise
1 to 2 tablespoons honey
1 teaspoon lemon juice
Poppy seeds to taste
1 tablespoon minced, crushed dill

Combine the white and red cabbage with the carrot. Add the red pepper, green pepper, and tomato. Whisk together the Nayonaise, honey, and lemon juice. Add the poppy seeds and dill. Toss with the vegetable mixture.

Halibut with Aunt Eunice's Marinade for Everything — Dinner

MAKES 3 CUPS

2 cups Dijon mustard

2 tablespoons crushed fresh garlic

1 tablespoon lemon pepper

2 teaspoons fine herb seasoning (or a combination of parsley, chervil, chives, and tarragon)

½ cup white or red wine vinegar, or a mixture of half fresh lemon juice and half vinegar

¼ cup extra virgin olive oil

⅓ cup light soy sauce

3 to 4 shakes hot sauce, optional

Red pepper flakes to taste, optional

4 6-ounce halibut steaks marinated in Aunt Eunice's Marinade for Everything

In a bowl (or blender), whisk together the mustard, garlic, lemon pepper, and fine herb. Add the vinegar, olive oil, soy sauce, and any optional flavorings. Marinate the steaks for 1 hour, covered, at room temperature. Broil or grill for 4 minutes on one side and approximately 6 minutes on the other.

Braised Bok Choy — Dinner

SERVES 4

1 tablespoon safflower oil

2 teaspoons minced garlic

1 large carrot, cut in scant ¼-inch diagonals, optional

1 teaspoon minced fresh ginger

1 cup sliced leek or scallions, cut in ½-inch diagonals

1 medium bok choy, cut in ½-inch diagonals, leaves coarsely chopped

1 cup rich vegetable stock

1 tablespoon tamari

Preheat the oven to 375 degrees. Heat a large, ovenproof skillet. Add the oil, garlic, and carrot and sauté for 1 minute, until the carrot begins to brown. Add the ginger and leek and sauté for 1 minute. Add the bok choy and sauté until slightly limp, a few seconds. Add the stock and tamari to the skillet and bring to a boil. Cover and place the skillet in the oven for 15 minutes. When done, simmer for 2 minutes longer on the stove to reduce the sauce, if necessary.

Legal Cheesecake — Dessert

SERVES 10

Crust

15 small graham crackers (try amaranth or oat bran)
3 tablespoons soy margarine, melted
½ teaspoon cinnamon or baking blend spice

Filling

5 cakes tofu (about 3½ pounds), coarsely crumbled
⅔ cup plain or flavored soy milk
¼ cup tahini
¾ cup maple syrup
2 egg whites
2 tablespoons fresh lemon juice
1½ teaspoons vanilla extract
Fresh fruit, such as grapes, apricots, cherries, or berries, optional

In a blender or food processor, crumble the graham crackers into coarse crumbs. Pour into an 8- or 9-inch springform pan and add the margarine and cinnamon. Stir well to combine and press firmly on the bottom of the pan.

Preheat the oven to 350 degrees. In a blender or food processor, puree the tofu in batches until smooth, adding about a tablespoon of soy milk with each batch. Scrape into a large bowl. Add the tahini, maple syrup, egg whites, lemon juice, and vanilla and stir well to combine.

Scrape into the prepared pan and smooth the top with a spatula. Bake for 30 minutes, until the filling is set and the top begins to turn golden. Cool on a rack, then cover and refrigerate until chilled. Before serving, remove the sides of the pan. Garnish with fresh fruit.

DAY 30

YELLOW WEEK

You made it! Tonight we're going to have a celebration dinner. Make it buffet style and have your friends over for that "recycle" party we talked about on Day 22, or make it an elegant sit-down dinner. (Just make sure to refer to my table seating theory on page 38 so that you know where to seat your friends.) Choose your dishes from the menu selections listed on the following pages and turn your friends on to your healthy new lifestyle. Who knows, you may end up with a new jacket, a convert, or an "anchor" in your life. (Review menu suggestions and create a personalized kitchen list, as you may not want to prepare all the dishes.)

MOTIVATIONAL TIP

There's that famous quote, **"THERE ARE TWO THINGS WE GIVE OUR CHILDREN. THE FIRST IS ROOTS; THE OTHER IS WINGS."** Hopefully these 30 days have given you the understanding and knowledge of what to do. After this week, you can go off and practice everything you've learned and create the rest of your life for yourself.

EXERCISE TIP

MAKE YOUR OWN FITNESS VIDEO. By this time you should have your own exercise program figured out. Have someone turn the camera on you, or set it up on a tripod

266

and film yourself as you're working out. Video is a great tool to evaluate the quality of your workout because you can check your form and style. If nothing else, it might be good for a laugh!

FOOD TIP

HOLD EVERYTHING! You're going to be ordering food in restaurants soon. The best way to get your food cooked the right way is to write down *exactly* what you *won't* eat on a piece of paper for the food server to take to the kitchen. For example, write down no dairy, no meat, no refined sugar, whatever you don't want in your food. This sounds demanding, but it's not. Restaurant owners recommend this. They don't want to serve you something that you will only send back to the kitchen. You can also tell them that you're allergic and will have a reaction. This always seems to work, especially if you don't feel your food server is being responsive!

ORGANIZATIONAL TIP

LONG-TERM ORGANIZATIONAL MAINTENANCE. We already talked about that "box," but maybe there are things around your house that still need work. (Hopefully it's not your sock drawer or your underwear drawer anymore.) Perhaps there are some curtains that need repair or lightbulbs that need to be changed. Whatever it is, on this final day, walk around your house and make a list of everything that still needs to be done. Maybe it'll take the next six months to do it all, but just cross off the tasks as you accomplish them. Write down anything that needs to be organized or fixed or cleaned, and keep that list handy.

BEAUTY TIP

FACE VALUE. In *Total Health Makeover*, I explained how to read your face for the telltale signs of bad eating. Now that you've been eating well for the last month, I will bet that your face has changed a great deal. The puffiness around your eyes and in your cheeks has probably gone down from the lack of dairy. The circles under your eyes have probably all but disappeared and/or changed colors. "Read" your face. If you still have a way to go, you might want to consider doing portions of the last month again.

SPA ON A BUDGET

SCRUB A DUB, DUB. Take 3 tablespoons of sea salt and ½ cup of almond oil and mix with water until it becomes a paste. Use it as a body scrub, but do not shave your legs before or after doing this. This is an inexpensive way of scrubbing your body head to toe—do it once a week or once a month.

TOTAL HEALTH FAKEOVER

BREAK A SWEAT EVERY DAY (PAS DE DEUX). You really don't need to fake it anymore, but if you do . . . We know we should break a sweat every day. From now on, if you really don't have time for exercise, you can take a really hot shower for at least ten minutes. You'll be amazed how much you sweat. Or you could always have at least ten minutes of really sweaty sex (preferably with a partner). It won't do much for your fitness level, but it will definitely give you a glow.

Menu

DAY 30

On Rising: 6 ounces fruit juice or 1 piece of fresh fruit

Breakfast: (2 hours after fruit) Pancakes

Lunch: Use your judgment (I trust you!)

Dinner: Dinner Party Buffet, your choice (depending on number of guests) from preceding recipes and/or any of the following: Mexican Pesto Dip, White Lotus Hummus, Trio of Olive Tapenade with Thyme and Garlic, Sunny Mustard Dill Sauce, Sunset Grill White Bean Salad, Black Beans with Chiles and Roasted Peppers, Mixed Greens with Herbed Sesame Dressing, Mushroom and Arugula Salad, Black Bean Dumplings, Winter Pasta from Along Came Mary, Salmon Tartare from the Aquagrill, Tofu Cakes with Coconut Cream and Two Salsas, Golden Crumble Cake. Just remember, don't *you* overdo it. (And be sure to be a swizzle stick!)

Pancakes — Breakfast

Buckwheat mix (follow directions on box)
Rice Dream (instead of milk)
Splash of vanilla
Dash of cinnamon
Soy margarine
Maple Syrup

Use any non-dairy pancake mix. Substitute Rice Dream for the milk and add vanilla and cinnamon to taste. Because it's Day 30, you can have a little bit of soy margarine and 100 percent maple syrup to celebrate.

White Lotus Hummus

8 ½-CUP SERVINGS

24-ounce jar Great Northern beans
2 tablespoons safflower oil
1 to 2 cloves garlic, minced
2 tablespoons umeboshi paste
¼ cup tahini
Juice of 1 lemon

In a blender or food processor, combine all the ingredients and puree until smooth. Scrape into a serving bowl and garnish with crackers, if desired.

Mexican Pesto Dip

SERVES 15

1 pound soft tofu

5 cloves garlic, peeled

1 jalapeño pepper, minced

1 bunch cilantro

2 tablespoons honey

2 tablespoons lemon juice

1 teaspoon salt

3 teaspoons ground cumin

½ pound jicama, sliced

1 red bell pepper, sliced

1 green pepper, sliced

Drain the tofu thoroughly and set aside. Fit a food processor with the metal chopping blade. With the motor running, drop the garlic and jalapeño into the processor bowl and process until minced. Remove. Cut the tough stems from the cilantro. Process the remaining cilantro leaves until finely minced. Add to the tofu mixture. Stir together the honey and lemon juice to dissolve. Add to the tofu mixture with the salt and cumin. Transfer the spread to a serving bowl or store in an airtight container until ready to serve. If spread is made ahead, drain liquid from edges before serving. Serve with jicama and pepper slices for dipping.

Trio of Olive Tapenade
with Thyme and Garlic

SERVES 15

Dale Greenblatt from Gourmet Fetishes tried and improved many of the recipes in this book. This is one of his own.

½ **pound black olives, sliced**
½ **pound green pimento-stuffed olives**
4 **ounces kalamata olives, pitted**
2 **large cloves garlic, minced**
3 **tablespoons minced fresh thyme**
½ **teaspoon crushed red pepper flakes**
¼ **teaspoon freshly ground white pepper**
2 **tablespoons fresh lemon juice**
¼ **cup extra virgin olive oil**

In a food processor fitted with a metal blade, pulse each of the olive varieties separately until minced, but not into a paste. Place the olive mixtures in a stainless steel bowl and mix well with the garlic, thyme, red pepper flakes, pepper, lemon juice, and olive oil. If necessary, adjust the seasonings with additional garlic, thyme, red pepper flakes, or lemon juice to taste. Serve with bread or toasts. Store refrigerated up to a week.

Dale Greenblatt
Gourmet Fetishes

Recipe

Sunny Mustard Dill Sauce

ABOUT 2 CUPS

1 10-ounce package soft tofu

2 teaspoons lemon juice

¼ cup soy milk

½ teaspoon pepper, cayenne if you like your food spicy

3 tablespoons melted soy margarine

¼ teaspoon honey

2 tablespoons natural mustard

3 tablespoons chopped fresh dill

In a blender or food processor, combine all the ingredients (in batches if necessary) and whirl for 30 seconds or until smooth.

Sunset Grill White Bean Salad over Mixed Greens and Miners Lettuce Finished with a Beet Vinaigrette

When I was on my book tour, I went to Nashville and ate at Sunset Grill. The chef, James Reesor, is young and talented and a real find!

Salad

4 cups Great Northern beans (soaked overnight)
1 cup diced avocado
1 cup diced plum tomatoes
1 cup diced red onions
1 cup diced roasted beets
3 tablespoons champagne vinegar
1 tablespoon julienned basil
Salt and pepper to taste

Vinaigrette

1 cup roasted beets
3 tablespoons raspberry vinegar
5 tablespoons red wine vinegar
3 tablespoons olive oil

Salad

Cook the beans until tender. Cool in the refrigerator. In a mixing bowl, combine all the ingredients and add salt and pepper to taste.

274

Vinaigrette

In a blender, blend the first 3 ingredients. Slowly add the olive oil, and salt and pepper if desired.

James Reesor
Chef, Sunset Grill, Nashville

Black Beans with Chiles and Roasted Peppers

SERVES 8

Here's a recipe from a dear friend of mine, Joe Rowley, who's an excellent chef. Watch for his cookbook, Some Recipes from a Couple Two, Tree Guys Dat Like to Cook, *coming soon.*

Once you've tasted this dish, two things will happen: First, you'll realize it is easily worth the effort, and second, your guests or family will crown you Cooking Genius of the Century. In short, it's sensational. Spicy, smoky, earthy, and rich are just a few of the adjectives that come to mind.

3 30-ounce cans black beans
1 yellow onion, finely chopped
Dried chiles arbol (flakes) to taste
Extra virgin olive oil
6 cloves garlic, smashed and finely chopped
3 red bell peppers, roasted, peeled, seeded, and chopped
3 poblano peppers, roasted, peeled, seeded, and chopped
3 jalapeño peppers, seeded and chopped (¼-inch dice)

3 serrano peppers, seeded and chopped (¼-inch dice)
½ cup finely chopped fresh cilantro
2 tablespoons ground cumin
Salt
Freshly ground black pepper

Strain the black beans, saving a cup or so of the liquid. (This will be used later for adjusting the consistency of the finished dish.)

Sauté the onion and chiles arbol in olive oil over medium heat until the onions wilt. Add the smashed garlic and cook for 2 to 3 minutes. Add the red bell, poblano, jalapeño, and serrano peppers along with a generous tablespoon of chopped cilantro. Sauté for 7 to 8 minutes, stirring frequently. The goal is to get the peppers to give up some of their water and allow the flavors to combine.

Stir the ground cumin, some salt, and a generous portion of freshly ground black pepper into the pepper and onion sauté. Add the beans and thoroughly mix it all together. Continue to cook over medium to low heat for 15 to 20 minutes. If the beans seem too dry, add a little of the water you saved when you strained the beans.

Taste and adjust the seasonings.

Spoon, ladle, or dump the beans into a large serving dish (a big pasta bowl is perfect) and garnish with a generous sprinkle of chopped cilantro. Now (with panache) carry the dish to the table, graciously acknowledging the applause and oohs and aahs.

Mixed Greens with Herbed Sesame Dressing

SERVES 4

3 tablespoons tahini

3 tablespoons lemon juice

1½ teaspoons umeboshi vinegar

3 cloves garlic, pressed or minced

1½ to 3 teaspoons minced fresh marjoram or ¾ to 1½ teaspoons dried

6 to 7 cups loosely packed mixed greens, torn into bite-sized pieces

1 to 2 cups finely sliced baby bok choy

4 scallions, finely minced

8 medium sorrel leaves, chopped or torn, optional

Lavender chive flowers, optional

Nasturtium blossoms, optional

In a small bowl, whisk together the tahini, lemon juice, vinegar, and garlic. Season with marjoram to taste. In a large bowl, toss together the greens, bok choy, scallions, and sorrel if desired. Divide among 4 plates. Drizzle dressing over each serving and garnish with chive flowers and nasturtiums if desired.

Mushroom and Arugula Salad (Insalata di Rucola con Funghi)

SERVES 4

This is my favorite salad from Coco Pazzo, one of my favorite restaurants in New York.

> **2 bunches arugula**
> **4 portobello mushroom caps, sliced**
> **6 ounces chanterelle mushrooms**
> **6 ounces hen of the woods (or any of your favorite) mushrooms**
> **¼ cup plus 1 teaspoon virgin olive oil**
> **4 tablespoons balsamic vinegar (aged, if possible)**
> **1 tablespoon finely chopped fresh rosemary**
> **1 tablespoon finely chopped fresh thyme**
> **1 tablespoon chopped fresh Italian parsley**
> **Salt**
> **Freshly ground black pepper**

Wash the arugula in warm water and dry. Cold water will damage the quality of the leaves. Clean all mushrooms with a wet cloth (do not wash the mushrooms in water because they will lose a lot of their flavor). For the balsamic vinaigrette, mix the ¼ cup olive oil, vinegar, and herbs together and season with salt. Set aside.

Arrange the arugula on a cold plate and set aside. Bring a pan to medium heat and add the 1 teaspoon olive oil and the mushrooms. Sauté lightly for about 1 minute and season with salt.

Place the hot mushrooms on the arugula and drizzle with balsamic vinaigrette. Finish with some freshly ground black pepper.

Black Bean Dumplings

YIELD: 12 DUMPLINGS

1 cup cooked black beans, mashed
¼ cup tahini (ground sesame seed)
1 ounce scallions, finely chopped
1 tablespoon tamari
1 tablespoon mirin
½ teaspoon rice wine vinegar
½ teaspoon ponzu (Japanese citrus)
Salt and ground pepper to taste
1 tablespoon chili garlic paste
12 dumpling skins (available at Asian markets)

Mix all the ingredients together in a bowl except for the dumpling skins. Put a drop of water around the edges of the dumpling skin. Add 1 teaspoon of black bean stuffing and seal tight. Sauté in a nonstick pan rubbed with olive oil. Brown 1 minute on each side. Finish in a 350-degree oven for 3 minutes.

Louis Lanza
Josie's Restaurant, New York

DAY 30

Winter Pasta from Along Came Mary

SERVES 4

My family is famous for its Christmas party, and this is a dish that the fabulous caterers from Along Came Mary cook every year. It's the number one request from our guests.

> **1 to 2 cloves garlic, minced**
> **Cooked white beans (see recipe below)**
> **4 tablespoons extra virgin olive oil**
> **4 bunches fresh spinach, washed, stemmed, and wilted**
> **2 tablespoons fresh thyme leaves, finely chopped**
> **1 tablespoon fresh basil leaves, finely chopped**
> **1 tablespoon oregano leaves, finely chopped**
> **½ cup to 1 cup reduced vegetable stock**
> **1 pound penne pasta, cooked al dente in salted water**
> **Salt**
> **Freshly ground black pepper**

Sauté the garlic and white beans in the olive oil. Add the spinach and herbs. Add the reduced stock and simmer 2 to 3 minutes. Add to the hot pasta and season with salt and black pepper.

Mary Micucci
Along Came Mary, Los Angeles

White Beans

1 pound dry white beans
1 carrot, peeled and cut into ¼-inch dice
2 stalks celery, washed and cut into ¼-inch dice
1 onion, peeled and cut into ¼-inch dice
2 cloves garlic, finely minced
¼ cup olive oil
2 sprigs thyme
1 bay leaf
6 sprigs parsley leaves
Salt
Freshly ground black pepper

Soak the beans overnight in cold water.

In a separate skillet, sauté the carrot, celery, onion, and garlic in the olive oil until just soft. Set aside. Put the presoaked beans in a large pot. Add enough fresh, cold water to cover by 2 inches. Slowly bring to a boil over low heat. Tie the thyme, bay leaf, and parsley together in a bouquet garni and add it to the pot, along with salt and black pepper. Turn down the heat to simmer and cook for 30 minutes. Add the vegetable mixture and cook for another 20 to 25 minutes, or until the beans are al dente. Remove the bouquet garni. Remove the beans from the heat and cool.

Salmon Tartare from the Aquagrill

SERVES 4 TO 6

My favorite dish in New York City! At Aquagrill, they serve salmon tartare as a complimentary hors d'oeuvre. The inspiration for this came from the classic steak tartare with the omission of egg yolks. It's a very easy and quick recipe. The most important aspect is to use fresh salmon.

> **1 pound salmon belly (or fillet), finely chopped**
> **Salt and freshly ground black pepper to taste**
> **⅛ cup chopped cornichon pickles**
> **⅛ cup chopped yellow onion**
> **⅛ cup capers**
> **2 tablespoons freshly chopped parsley**
> **2 tablespoons freshly chopped chives**
> **6 tablespoons Dijon mustard**

Season the fish by sprinkling lightly with salt and pepper. Add all the ingredients except 1 tablespoon of chives. Combine without mashing. Chill 30 minutes to set the flavors. Sprinkle with the remaining chives.

Jeremy Marshall
Aquagrill, New York

Tofu Cakes with Coconut Cream and Two Salsas

Avalon of Maui is one of the premier restaurants in Hawaii. The food is great and the chef, Mark Ellman, is a wonderful guy.

- 6 ounces fresh tofu, firm and strained of any extra moisture
- ¼ cup seasoned panko flakes (Japanese bread crumbs; available at Asian markets)
- ⅛ cup minced scallions
- 1 teaspoon chopped fresh ginger
- 1 teaspoon chopped fresh garlic
- 1 teaspoon chopped fresh mint
- 1 teaspoon chopped fresh basil
- 1 teaspoon chopped fresh cilantro
- ⅛ cup chili sauce
- 1 teaspoon Hawaiian salt
- 1 cup seasoned panko flakes with Hawaiian salt and pepper
- ⅜ cup olive oil
- ¾ cup coconut cream
- 1 tablespoon mango salsa
- 1 tablespoon tomato salsa

In a bowl, mash the tofu very fine. Add the remaining ingredients through the salt and mix gently. Form into patties and roll in the seasoned panko flakes. Chill for 2 hours.

In a non-stick pan, sauté the patties in the olive oil until golden on each side. Place in a 400-degree oven for 10 to 15 minutes.

To make the coconut cream, in a sauté pan, reduce 2 cups of coconut milk with 1 tablespoon chopped ginger, 1 teaspoon low-sodium soy sauce, 1 chopped fresh lemongrass stalk, 2 kaffir lime leaves, 2 basil stems, 2 mint stems, and 2 cilantro stems, by half, or until viscous. Strain and leave at room temperature.

Lace the coconut cream on the plate in a circle, place the cakes on top of the sauce, and top each cake with salsa—one with mango, the other with tomato. For garnish, from a squeeze bottle, zigzag hoisin sauce around the cakes. Top with toasted sesame seeds and fresh cilantro leaves.

Mango Salsa

1 mango or papaya or pineapple, diced small
¼ Maui onion, diced small
3 tablespoons freshly chopped mint
⅛ cup lime juice
Salt and pepper to taste

Mix all the ingredients in a bowl at least 1 hour before serving.

Tomato Salsa

1 tomato, diced small
¼ Maui onion, diced small
3 tablespoons chopped cilantro
⅛ cup lime juice
¼ cup of macadamia nut oil
2 tablespoons capers
Salt and pepper to taste

Mix all the ingredients in a bowl at least 1 hour before serving.

Chef Mark Ellman
Avalon of Maui

284

Golden Crumble Cake

SERVES 8

Cake

    ½ **cup soy margarine**
    2 **tablespoons maple syrup or honey**
    2 **eggs**
    ½ **cup soy yogurt**
    1 **14-ounce package oatmeal raisin cookie mix**

Topping

    2 **teaspoons soy margarine, melted**
    ⅓ **cup maple syrup or honey**
    ½ **cup chopped pecans or walnuts**
    ⅓ **cup raspberry granola**

Preheat the oven to 350 degrees. In a mixing bowl, cream the margarine, maple syrup, eggs, and soy yogurt. Blend in the cookie mix, adding a tablespoon or two of water if necessary to bind the dough. Spread into a lightly greased 8-inch or 9-inch pan. Bake for 35 minutes, or until light gold. Preheat the broiler. Combine the topping ingredients and distribute evenly over the warm cake. Broil for about 2 minutes, until the top is glossy and golden.

Appendix
Marilu's Pantry Stockers

This is a partial list of the many different foods and brands that I've used and approved. If you can't find them in your local natural food store, you might want to look for the companies (and their mail-order policies) on the Internet.

Cold Cereals

1. Arrowhead Mills: Wheat Flakes, Bran Flakes, Oat Bran Flakes, Corn Flakes, Puffed Wheat, Puffed Rice, Puffed Millet, Puffed Corn, Nature O's, Amaranth Flakes, Spelt Flakes, Kamut, Multigrain Flakes

2. Barbara's Bakery: Corn Flakes, Breakfast O's, Brown Rice Crisps, Shredded Wheat, Shredded Spoonfuls, High 5, Raisin Bran, Breakfast Biscuits

3. Health Valley: Honey Clusters and Flakes: Apple Cinnamon, Honey Crunch; Organic Bran Cereal with Raisins, 100% Natural Bran Cereal with Apples and Cinnamon, Real Oat Bran Cereal-Almond Flavored Crunch, Organic Healthy Fiber Multi-Grain Flakes, Organic Blue Corn Flakes, Organic Oat Bran Flakes with Raisins, Organic Fiber 7 Flakes, Organic Amaranth Flakes, Organic Oat Bran Flakes, Organic Raisin Bran Flakes, Oat Bran O's, Stone Wheat Flakes, Fat-Free Granola

4. Kellogg Company: Nutri-Grain: Corn, Wheat, Nuggets, and so on

5. Kolln: Oat Bran Crunch

6. Nabisco: Shredded Wheat

7. Perky Foods: Crispy Brown Rice, Nutty Rice

8. Post: Grape-Nuts

9. U.S. Mills: Erewhon: Wheat Flakes, Kamut Flakes, Aztec, Super-O's, Corn Flakes, Raisin Grahams, Honey Crisp Corn, Galaxy Grahams, Apple Strudels, Banana O's, Skinner's Raisin Bran, Skinner's Low Sodium Raisin Bran, Uncle Sam Cereal

10. Weetabix Company: Grainfields: Wheat Flakes, Corn Flakes, Raisin Bran, Wheetabix Whole Wheat Cereal

Hot Cereals

1. Arrowhead Mills: Instant Oatmeal, Maple Apple Spice, Original Plain, Bear Mush, Cracked Wheat, 7 Grain, Oat Bran

2. Barbara's Bakery: 14 Grains

3. Kashi Company: Kashi

4. Lundberg Family Farms: Hot 'N Creamy Rice Cereals: Cinnamon Raisin, Amber Grain

5. Pritikin Systems: Hearty Hot Cereal, Apple Raisin Spice

6. Quaker Oats Company: Quaker Oats, Quick Quaker Oats

7. Stone Ground Mills, Inc.: 7-Grain Cereal, Cracked Wheat Cereal, Hot Apple Granola, Scotch Oats, Old Fashioned Rolled Oats

8. U.S. Mills: Skinner's Oat Bran, Skinner's Toasted Oat Rings; Erewhon: Barley Plus, Brown Rice Cream, Oat Bran with Toasted Wheat Germ, Apple Cinnamon Oatmeal, Apple Raisin Oatmeal, Maple Spice Oatmeal, Dates and Walnuts Oatmeal, Oatmeal with Added Oatbran

Acceptable Milk Substitutes

1. American Natural Snacks: Harmony Farms: Fat-Free Rice Drink, Soya Kaas Cream Cheese Style Spread

2. Chino Valley: Veg-a-Fed Cage Fed Large Eggs

3. Eden Foods: Eden Rice Beverage, Edensoy Vanilla Soy Milk

4. Galaxy Foods: Veggie Slices

5. Grainaissance: Amazake Rice Drink, Amazake Light

6. Health Valley Foods: Soy Moo (low-fat), Fat-Free Soy Moo

7. Imagine Foods: Rice Dream: Original, Vanilla, Carob, Chocolate, Original Enriched, Vanilla Enriched, Carob Enriched, Chocolate Enriched, Non-dairy frozen desserts, assorted flavors. Soy Dream: Original, Vanilla, Carob, Chocolate, Original Enriched, Vanilla Enriched, Carob Enriched, Chocolate Enriched

8. Pacific Foods of Oregon: Pacific Lite

9. Soyco Foods: Lite & Less Grated Parmesan Cheese Alternative, Low-fat Rice Cream Cheese Style, Rice Slice: American, Mozzarella, and Swiss

10. Turtle Mountain, Inc.: Sweet Nothings Non-Dairy Frozen Desserts, assorted flavors

11. Vitasoy USA: Vitasoy Light-Original 1%

12. Westbrae Natural Foods: Non Fat West Soy Milk, West Soy Lite (1% Fat) Plain

13. White Wave: Silk (1% Fat) Non-dairy Yogurt, various flavors

Hot Drinks

1. Bioforce of America: Coffree, Bambu

2. California Natural Products: Dacopa

3. Eden Foods: Yannoh

4. General Foods Corp: Postum

5. Libby, McNeil, & Libby: Pero

6. Many manufacturers: Herbal teas

7. Richter Bros: Cafix

8. Worthington Foods: Kaffree Roma

Soy Sauces

1. Edward & Sons Trading Company: Ginger Tamari

2. Kikkoman Foods: Kikkoman Lite Soy Sauce

3. Live Food Products: Bragg's Liquid Aminos (used often in recipes; please buy)

4. San-J International: Tamari Wheat Free Soy Sauce

5. Westbrae Natural Foods: Mild Soy Sauce

Salad Dressings

1. American Health Products: El Molino Herbal Secrets

2. Annie's: Wild-Herbal Organics, Green Garlic Vinaigrette

3. Ayla's Organics: Oil Free: many varieties; Russian Fat-free Salad Dressing

4. Cardini's: Select Italian Dressing

5. Consorzio's: Vignette Mustard Seed Flavored Vinegar

6. Cook's Classics: Cook's Classics Oil Free Dressings: Italian Gusto, Country French, Garlic Gusto, Dijon, Dill

7. Hain Pure Foods: Fat Free Salad Dressing Mix: Italian, Herb

8. Kozlowski Farms: Fat-free Dressings: Zesty Herb, Honey Mustard, South of the Border, Raspberry Poppy Seed

9. Nakano USA: Seasoned Rice Vinegar

10. Nature's Harvest: Oil-Free Vinaigrette, Oil-Free Herbal Splendor

11. Newman's Own: Various dressings (make sure they're non-dairy)

12. Pritikin Systems: No Oil Dressing: Tomato, Italian, Russian, Creamy Italian, etc.

13. Rising Sun Farms, Inc.: Oil Free Salad Vinaigrettes and Marinades: Raspberry Balsamic, Garlic Lovers, Dill with Lemon, Honey & Mustard

14. S&W Fine Foods: Vintage Lites Oil-Free Dressing

15. Sweet Adelaide Enterprises: Paula's No-Oil Dressing: Toasted Onion, Roasted Garlic, Garden Tomato, Lime and Cilantro, Lemon Dill

16. The Mayhaw Tree: Vidalia Onion Vinegar

17. Tres Classique: Grand Garlic, Tomato & Herb French Dressing

18. Uncle Grant's Foods: Uncle Grant's Salute-Honey Mustard Taragon Dressing

19. Simply Delicious: Miso Sesame, other varieties

20. Tree of Life: Italian Garlic, assorted fat-free dressings

21. W.M. Reilly & Company: Herb Magic: Vinaigrette, Italian, Gypsy, Zesty Tomato

Other Sauces and Pastes

1. American Miso Co.: Miso Master various miso flavors

2. Annie Chun's Gourmet Foods: Fat Free Mushroom Sauce, Oil Free Teriyaki Sauce

3. Ayla's Organics: Cajun, Curry, Szechwan, Thai Sauce

4. Durkee-French Foods: Red Hot Sauce

5. Edward & Sons Trading Company: Stir Crazy Vegetarian Worcestershire Sauce

6. Enrico's: Assorted tomato sauces

7. Gourmet Foods: Cajun Sunshine

8. J. Sosnick & Son: Kosher Horseradish

9. Lang Naturals, Inc.: Fat Free Sauces: Honey Mustard, Ginger, Tangy Bang! Hot Sauce, Garlic Steak Sauce, Thai Peanut Sauce, Ginger Stir-Fry Sauce, Honey Mustard Sauce, Sweet & Sour Sauce, Indian Curry Sauce

10. Mama Coco's: Assorted tomato sauces (make sure they're non-dairy)

11. New Morning: Corn Relish

12. Oak Hill Farms: Vidalia Onion Steak Sauce, Three Pepper Lemon Hot Sauce

13. Organic Gourmet: Miso Paste: Honey, Apple

14. Reese Finer Foods: Prepared Horseradish, Old English Tavern Sauce

15. St. Giles Foods, Ltd: Matured Worcestershire Sauce

16. Whole Foods: Assorted tomato sauces

Seasoning Mixtures

1. Alberto-Culver Company: Mrs. Dash; Low Pepper–No Garlic, Extra Spicy, Original Blend, etc.

2. Barth's Nutrafoods: NutraSoup: Vegetable

3. Bernard Jensen Products: Broth or Seasoning Special Vegetable Mix

4. Estee Corp: Seasoning Sense: Mexican, Italian

5. Hain Pure Food Company: Chili Seasoning Mix

6. Maine Coast Sea Vegetables: Sea Seasonings: Dulse with Garlic, Nori with Ginger, etc.

7. Modern Products: Vegit All-Purpose Seasoning, Onion Magic, Natural Seasoning, Herbal Bouquet, Garlic Magic

8. Parsley Patch: All Purpose, Mexican Blend

Soups: Dry Packaged

1. AFC Corp: Natural Tofu Miso Soup

2. Eden Foods: Ramen: Buckwheat, Whole Wheat

3. Fantastic Foods: Rice & Beans, Five Bean Soup, Cha-Cha Chili, Vegetable, Barley, Couscous with Lentils, Country Lentil, Black Bean Salsa Couscous, Pinto Beans and Rice Mexicana; Ramen Noodles: Chicken-Free, Tomato, Vegetable Curry, Miso

4. Health Valley Foods: Pasta Italiano, Fat-Free Cup of Soup-Marinara, Garden Split Pea with Carrots, Spicy Black Bean with Couscous, Zesty Black Bean with Rice, Chicken Flavored Noodles with Vegetables, Lentil with Couscous

5. Nile Spice Foods: Lentil Soup, Black Bean Soup, Split Pea Soup, Chili 'N Beans; Pack It Meals: Black Bean, Red Beans and Rice, Lentil Curry

6. Pacific Foods of Oregon: Chef's Classics: Caribbean Black Beans and Rice, Savory Lentil, Minestrone, Cajun Red Beans & Rice, Curried Lentils & Rice

7. Sahara Natural Foods: Casbah: Hearty Harvest, Original Couscous, Jambalaya, Moroccan Stew, La Fiesta

8. Sokensha Company: Soken Ramen

9. The Spice Hunter: Moroccan Couscous, Mediterranean Minestrone, Cantonese Noodle Soup, French Country Lentil, Kasba Curry, Kasba Curry with Rice Bran, Mandarin Noodle Soup

10. Trader Joe's: Ramen Soup, Brown Rice Ramen, Soba Noodles

11. U.S. Mills: Erewhon Japanese Misos: Genmai Miso, Kome Miso, Hatcho Miso, Mugi Miso

12. Westbrae Natural Foods: Ramen: Whole Wheat, Onion, Curry, Carrot, Miso, Seaweed, 5-Spice, Spinach, Mushroom, Buckwheat, Savory Szechwan, Oriental Vegetable, Golden Chinese; Instant Miso Soup: Mellow White, Hearty Red; Noodles Anytime—Country Style

13. Wil-Pak Foods: Taste Adventure Foods: Black Bean, Curry Lentil, Split Pea, Red Bean, Navy Bean, Minestrone, Red Bean Chili, Black Bean Chili, Lentil Chili, 5 Bean Chili

14. W.M. Reilly & Company: Bean Cuisine Soup

Soups: Canned

1. Fair Exchange, Inc.: Shari's Bistro Soups: Tomato with Roasted Garlic, Great Plains Split Pea, Indian Black Beans and Rice, Spicy French Green Lentil, Mexican Bean Burrito Soup/Dip

2. Hain Pure Food Company: Fat-Free Soup: Vegetarian Split Pea, Vegetarian Veggie Broth

3. Health Valley Foods: Organic Potato Leek Soup, Organic Mushroom Barley Soup, Organic Black Bean Soup, Organic Split Pea Soup, Organic Minestrone Soup, Organic Lentil Soup; Fat-Free Soups: 14 Garden Vegetable Soup, Vegetable Barley, Country; Corn & Vegetable, 5 Bean Vegetable, Vegetable Soup, Tomato Vegetable, Split Pea & Carrots, Lentil & Carrots, Black Bean & Vegetable; Fat-Free Carotene Soups: Italian Plus, Super Broccoli, Vegetable Power; Organic Soups: Mushroom Barley, Potato Leek, Tomato, Black Bean, Split Pea, Minestrone, Vegetable

4. Little Bear Organic: Bearitos fat-free soups

5. Mercantile Food Company: American Prairie Vegetable Bean Soup

6. Muir Glen: Organic Tomato Soup

7. Pritikin Systems, Inc.: Vegetable Broth, Vegetarian Vegetable

8. Westbrae Natural Foods: Fat Free Soups of the World: Great Plains Savory Bean, Santa Fe Vegetable, Louisiana Bean Stew, Alabama Black Bean Gumbo, Old World Split Pea, Spicy Southwest Vegetable, Rich Mediterranean Lentil

Dry Packaged Grains and Pastas

1. Arrowhead Mills: Wholegrain Teff, Wheat-Free Oatbran Muffin Mix, Griddle Lite Pancake and Baking Mix; Quick Brown Rice: Spanish Style, Vegetable Herb, Wild Rice and Herbs, Whole Wheat Flour

2. Aurora Import & Dist: Polenta

3. Continental Mills: Ala-Cracked Wheat Bulgur

4. Fantastic Foods: Rice: Brown Basmati Rice, Plain, Brown Jasmine; Couscous, Whole Wheat Couscous; Quick Pilaf: Savory Couscous, Brown Rice with Miso, Spanish Brown Rice, Three Grain with Herbs

5. Jerusalem Natural Foods: Jerusalem Tab-ooleh

6. Liberty Imports: Instant Polenta

7. Lundberg Family Farms: One-Step Entrees: Chili, Curry, Basil; Rizcous, Quick Spanish Fiesta Pilaf, Quick Brown Rice

8. Near East Food Prod: Spanish Rice, Wheat Pilaf, Taboule, Lentil Pilaf Mix

9. Nile Spice Foods: Whole Wheat Couscous, Couscous Salad Mix, Rozdali

10. Pritikin Systems: Mexican Dinner Mix, Brown Rice Pilaf

11. Quinoa Corp: Quinoa

12. Sahara Natural Foods: Casbah Timeless Pilafs: Couscous, Lentil, Spanish, Bulgur, Wheat

13. San Gennaro Foods, Inc.: Polenta

14. Sorrenti Family Farms: Rising Star Ranch: Fiesta Rice, Harvest Rice, Pasta Roma

15. Texmati Rice: Basmati Brown Rice

16. The Food Merchants: Kamut Pasta Pilaf Southwestern Blend

17. Trader Joe's: Santa Fe Rice, Creole Rice, Spanish Rice

18. Wil-Pak Foods: Taste Adventure: Black Bean Flakes, Pinto Bean Flakes

19. W.M. Reilly & Company: Pasta and Beans

20. Worthington Foods: Natural Touch Taco Mix

Sodas

1. R.W. Knudsen: All Natural Carbonated Juices: assorted flavors

Juices

1. R.W. Knudsen: Assorted Organic Juices, Spritzers

2. Ferraros: Earth Juice, Mango Me, Orange Carrot, and assorted flavors

Condiments

1. Cascadian Farms: Sweet Relish and other organic assorted pickles and relishes, sauerkraut

2. Follow Your Heart: Vegenaise

3. Nasoya Foods, Inc.: Nayonaise, Vegi Dressing and Spread

4. Organic Foods Products: Millina's Finest assorted flavors, Pasta Sauces, Crushed Garlic

5. Organic Gourmet: Organic Gourmet Instant Soup-n-Stock Vegetable Concentrate

6. Shady Maple Farms: 100% Maple Syrup

7. Sorrel Ridge: Sorrel Ridge Jams: assorted flavors

8. Westbrae Natural Foods: Fruit Sweetened Catsup, Yellow Mustard

Desserts/Snacks

1. Imagine Foods: Puddings: assorted flavors, Non-dairy Rice Dream, Non-Dairy Frozen Desserts

2. Pavich: Organically Grown Raisins

3. Oy Panda Ab: Panda Licorice: assorted flavors

4. Hains Foods: Rice Cakes: Assorted flavors and snack sizes, Graham Crackers: assorted flavors

5. R.W. Frookies, Inc.: Frookwich Sandwich Cookies, sweetened with fruit juices: assorted flavors

6. Kettle Chips: Kettle Chips Potato Chips: Assorted flavors, all natural

7. Lundberg Family Farms: Lundberg Organic Rice Cakes

8. Guiltless Gourmet: Corn Chips

9. Auburn Farms: Toast-n-Jammers

Meat Substitutes

1. Lightlife Foods, Inc.: Smart Deli Meatless Slices: turkey, chicken, pepperoni, assorted flavored meat substitutes

2. Lightlife: Tofu Pups 100% Smart Dogs, Fat Free Vegi Hot Dogs

3. Yves Five Foods: Yves Veggie Breakfast Links

4. Boca-Burger, Inc.: Boca Burger Vegan Original Non-Dairy, Eggless, Meatless Burgers

Frozen Vegetables

1. Cascadian Farms: Green Peas, Corn, Green Beans, Carrots, French Fries

2. Edamame: Soybeans

Spreads

1. Shedd's Willow Run: Soy Margarine 100% Soybean Oil

2. American Natural Snacks: Soya Kaas Cream Cheese Style Spread

3. Soyco Foods: Rice Cream Cheese Style Spread, low-fat, non-dairy

Frozen Foods

1. Natural Sea: Fish sticks whole grain breaded, Fish Fillets

2. Amy's Kitchen, Inc.: Tofu Lasagna and assorted meals and TV dinners

3. Gloria's Kitchen: Tofu Balls with Organic Spaghetti

4. Health and Wealth Products: Chicken Nuggets, Stone Ground Whole Wheat Bread; White Chicken Patties, Chicken Free Patties, Tofu Munchies, Pizza, Spinach

5. Melrose Made Gourmet: Broccoli Souffle, Zucchini Souffle, Vegetable Souffle

6. Mon Cuisine: Vegetarian Salisbury Steak, Vegetarian Breaded Chicken Style Cutlet, Vegetarian Stuffed Cabbage

7. Vans: Non-Dairy, Eggless, Yeast and Gluten Free Toaster Waffles

8. Worthington Foods, Inc.: Natural Touch Burgers, Okara Patties, Natural Touch Lentil Rice Loaf

9. Northern Soy: Soy Boy Ravioli, Non-dairy, Organic Tofu

10. Celentano Bros: Celentano Non-Dairy Vegetarian Selects, Manicotti and assorted dishes

Breads
1. Food For Life: Ezekiel 4:9 Whole Wheat, Cinnamon Raisin

Cuisine Spices
1. Modern Products, Inc: Spike All Natural Seasoning, Vege-Sal All-Purpose Vegetized Seasoning, Spice Garden assorted spices

2. Whole Foods Brand: Assorted spices

3. Frontier Herbs: Non-irradiated assorted spices

4. Desert Spice: All Purpose Bedouin Seasoning

Mexican
Fresh cilantro, fresh green onion, fresh bell pepper, fresh limes, cumin, jalapeño pepper flakes, Mexican oregano

Italian
Tarragon, basil, garlic, pine nuts, extra virgin olive oil, fennel, thyme, Italian parsley, rosemary, balsamic vinegar, sun-dried tomatoes

Chinese
Five spice, soy sauce, any Chinese rice wine vinegar, fresh ginger

Indian
Curry, cayenne, cardamom, garlic masala, turmeric, cinnamon, tahini

Japanese
Mirin, rice vinegar, soy sauce different variations, miso, ginger, sesame oil, sesame seeds, nori

Books by Marilu Henner

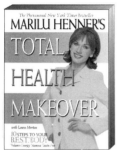

MARILU HENNER'S TOTAL HEALTH MAKEOVER
ISBN 0-06-098878-9 (paperback); ISBN 0-06-039216-9 (hardcover)
ISBN 0-06-109828-0 (mass market); ISBN 0-694-51927-8 (audio)

With irrepressible enthusiasm and humor, Marilu presents practical advice on diet myths, toxic foods, mood swings, food combining, and her unique, flexible, down-to-earth 10-step life plan. With *Marilu Henner's Total Health Makeover* you can free yourself from diets and disease-causing toxins, boost your energy, lower and maintain your weight, and change your outlook in as little as three weeks.

THE 30-DAY TOTAL HEALTH MAKEOVER
Everything You Need to Do to Change Your Body,
Your Health, and Your Life in 30 Amazing Days
ISBN 0-06-103133-X (paperback); ISBN 0-06-039291-6 (hardcover)

This inspirational how-to guide for total health living includes day-to-day goals; strategies for success; recipes for breakfast, lunch, and dinner; shopping lists; exercise ideas; and what to feed the kids. This concise and efficient plan to your B.E.S.T. body on your terms is for anyone who wants to look and feel great in just 30 days.

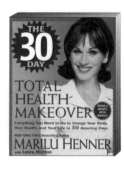

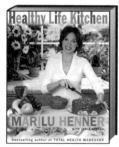

HEALTHY LIFE KITCHEN
ISBN 0-06-039364-5 (hardcover)

Marilu Henner provides a delicious collection of healthy recipes that will help readers change their bodies and their lives forever. Created by Marilu and her favorite chefs from restaurants all over the world, these delectable breakfasts, lunches, dinners, desserts, and snacks will bring healthy cuisine to a new level of taste and ease. The cookbook also contains a "healthy junkfood" section for converting the naughty treats you crave into nutritious recipes you can enjoy anytime.

I REFUSE TO RAISE A BRAT
ISBN 0-06-098730-8 (paperback); ISBN 0-694-52129-9 (audio)

Super-mom Marilu Henner and renowned psychoanalyst Dr. Ruth Sharon provide simple and straightforward advice on how to raise secure, happy and self-reliant children. *I Refuse to Raise a Brat* teaches readers how to distinguish between overgratification and love, break the pattern of overindulgence, and offer children the balance of frustration and gratification they need.

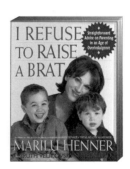

Available wherever books are sold, or call 1-800-331-3761 to order.